PRAISE FOR *DIET-PROOF*

Diet-Proof Your Daughter is a clear, kind, and reassuring guide for any parent who is worried about their child's relationship to food and body—but also still reckoning with the ways diet culture harms us all. Sherry encourages us to trust our daughters and in doing so, gives us the tools to begin to rebuild trust with ourselves.

—Virginia Sole-Smith, author of *Fat Talk: Parenting in the Age of Diet Culture* and the Burnt Toast Newsletter

Diet Proof Your Daughter is a must-have book for mothers looking to instill body and food confidence in their daughter in today's very complicated diet culture landscape. Amelia Sherry has a beautiful gift with words, sharing anecdotes with science, making this book powerful to read and easy to understand.

—Wendy Sterling, MS, RD, CSSD, CEDRDS, co-author, *Raising Body Positive Teens*

Any daughter would be lucky to have a mother who reads this book! Diet-Proof is for any mother contemplating taking an anti-diet stance in her family life—no matter where she is on her own healing journey. Sherry's relatable, personal story and thoughtful, reflection questions woven throughout create ample space for ambivalent readers to feel understood and inspired to break the toxic cycle of generational food and body shame.

—Zoë Bisbing, licensed psychotherapist, founder of Body-Positive NYC and The Full Bloom Project, a body-positive parenting resource

As a pediatrician, a mother, and a reformed chronic dieter this book is the language of my life. If every human that interacted with girls and young women acted on Amelia's advice we would be living in a healed and much happier world.

—Maggie Landes, MD, MPH, pediatrician, HAES® health-care educator, and host of the Health Can't Weight podcast

Now more than ever, parents need *Diet-Proof Your Daughter*. Amelia lays out—step by step—how parents can help their daughters avoid dieting and weight-centric pitfalls, building a solid foundation for health that will last a lifetime. This is a must-read for every parent of girls!

—Maryann Jacobsen, MS, RD, author of *My Body's Superpower: The Girls' Guide to Growing Up Healthy During Puberty*

Breaking intergenerational cycles of disordered eating and body shame isn't easy, especially in a world that bombards us with harmful messages about food and appearance. With this go-to guide, mothers now have the essential information and tools to protect their daughters from diet culture's threats to their self-image and well-being.

—Oona Hanson, nationally-recognized parent coach, advocate for eating disorder prevention, and founder of *Parenting Without Diet Culture*

Shining a bright light for mothers of daughters, including real-life stories, personal experiences, and professional guidance, Amelia Sherry helps modern-day moms navigate diet culture and its influence on their growing girls. If you have a daughter, this is a must-read!

—Jill Castle, MS, RDN, Founder of The Nourished Child® and author of *Size Wise* (Workman, 2023), *Eat Like a Champion*, and co-author of *Fearless Feeding*

DIET-PROOF YOUR DAUGHTER

DIET-PROOF YOUR DAUGHTER

A MOTHER'S GUIDE TO RAISING GIRLS WHO HAVE HAPPY, HEALTHY RELATIONSHIPS WITH FOOD AND BODY

AMELIA SHERRY, MPH, RD, CDCES

AS Nutrition Publishing
NEW YORK

To my darling Isla, who took me from disheartened to inspired with nothing but a few sweet breaths.

And to all the mothers who are wondering about the right thing to do. You are the right thing. Keep doing it.

Diet-Proof Your Daughter
Copyright © 2022 Amelia Sherry

ISBN: 979-8-218-13069-5 (hardcover)
ISBN 979-8-218-09118-7 (paperback)
ISBN 979-8-218-09119-4 (ebook)
Library of Congress Control Number 2022919648

Cover Design by Heather VenHuizen
Text Design by Streetlight Graphics
Author Photograph by Abby Greenawalt

First Printing 2022

AS Nutrition Publishing
Hastings-on-Hudson, New York
amelia@ameliasherry.com

TABLE OF CONTENTS

INTRODUCTION

W HEN I FOUND OUT MY FIRST CHILD WAS A GIRL, I SOBBED.
To be clear, these weren't tears of joy. These were tears of dread and fear and not wanting. Mostly dread. Aside from my husband, I'm not sure anyone knew just how much I'd been wishing, hoping, and praying to mother a boy. I felt that way not just during my pregnancy but before it, when our child was still just a hypothetical, dancing around in conversations over dinner. I was too ashamed of my boy-longing to contemplate what was behind it. And to make it easy on everyone, I stayed silent and privately sure, very sure, that I would be mothering a 'he.' When that sureness finally broke and my OB held my daughter in the air for me to see, I let out waves of despair. The emotion felt as confusing and frightening as it did shameful. And it'd take me almost a decade before I'd have the courage to dredge it back up to figure out its meaning.

Don't worry! The story's happy ending comes much sooner than that. Within 15 minutes of that first sighting, my daughter sent me into the deepest awe; I held her newborn skin against my own and watched her nurse. In her nursing, I saw the purest form of knowing. It reassured me in the deepest of deep; it comforted me and connected me to something more powerful than fear. For many years afterward, that sobbing seemed irrelevant and ridiculous, and it was practically forgotten.

As I write this, I can hear both of my daughters—now ten and six years old—banging around the house, scrambling for those shoes and gloves and hats that have been tucked and lost and tripped over. They're readying themselves to head out on a cold December day in New York.

1

My oldest is asking her father questions about the weather, the wind, the precipitation, all so she can strategize which pants to wear for their hike. As I listen to her voice, I know for sure it's important to remember the dread, fear, and sobbing. And it's more important to wonder out loud why, in 2011, a 36-year-old woman living in the western world would fall apart in fear and dread at the news that she'd just become a mother to a healthy baby girl.

Today, I now know that I wasn't so much longing to raise a boy as I was terrified of mothering a girl. To me, mothering a girl meant shepherding another young someone through the pain, doubt, and self-loathing which seemed an inevitable part of living in and managing a female body. And for me, those feelings I had buried started to well up and resurface just as my beautiful first child was approaching puberty and mostly when we came together at the table to eat.

FROM MOTHER TO DAUGHTER

Every mom wants her daughter to have a happy, healthy relationship with food. We want this for daughters because it's the thing we wish for ourselves, too: to be able to eat until we are full and satisfied, to stop counting calories and analyzing nutrition labels, to stop worrying that our friends and family members are judging us, and to stop judging ourselves. And yet, our diet-obsessed, photoshopped models, Instagram-perfect culture puts a laser focus on women's bodies and, therefore, women's eating. This pressure creates a constant internal struggle that most women know all too well. This struggle leads us to focus on our weight and inevitably shows up in our relationship with food, meal after meal. As a nutritionist who has worked with hundreds of mother and daughter pairs, I know we stand on potent ground when we start conversations about what we are eating and not eating, how much we are eating and not eating, and how we regard our unique shape, size, and weight.

As a new mom to a girl, I was petrified of watching my own daughter suffer from the needless worry, judgment, pressure, and tension that

I myself have felt throughout most of my life when it came to my body and eating. Today, I want nothing more than to give my girls—and all the girls I have the honor of working with—something so few women have ever had. I want to give them permission to have a peaceful relationship with food. I want to help them have a natural ease about eating and a matter-of-factness about nutrition. I want to help them have a positive approach to movement, and a deep and constant appreciation of their ever-changing bodies, be they large, small, or anything in between. And if they one day decide to become mothers, I want them to have nothing to fear when it comes to mothering their own girls in the realms of food, eating, movement, and weight.

If that's something that you want for the girls in your life, too, then my friend, this book is for you. If you picked up this book hoping for lists of nutritious foods with quantities and serving sizes for growing girls, please put it down immediately. Sorry–not sorry; but you won't find that here.

If you picked up this book because you regret all the hours, days, weeks, months, years, or even decades that you've spent worrying about what and how much to eat, and because now you want nothing more than to protect your own daughter(s) from a similar fate, then stay—we have something to talk about.

You might be thinking, what kind of nutritionist invites you to stop worrying about what your daughter *eats*? Isn't it our job as mothers to worry about what our kids eat and don't eat? Well, yes and no. Mostly no. It's our job to provide food for our children on a regular basis, yes. It's our job to do our best to make sure those meals are safe, edible, and nourishing, yes. But it's *not* our job to worry and wonder, to stress and fret about everything they eat and don't eat. And I want to convince you of that. Feeling relaxed about your daughter's eating is paramount when it comes to raising a healthy, happy, and well-nourished human. I not only believe that wholeheartedly, I have an abundance of proof to help you understand why. You'll find it throughout this book. Having a calm and trusting approach towards eating and body size, shape, and weight is of premier importance when it comes to raising a daughter who is diet-proof, or, in other words, a happy, healthy, and well-adjusted eater.

THERE'S A BETTER WAY

Like so many women, I have spent decades dieting and wasting time obsessing about the results those diets have had on my body and my weight. On top of that, I've also spent years writing articles on similar topics for women's magazines, then counseling patients and clients as a nutrition professional on which foods to eat and to avoid to achieve "a better body," "optimal health," and "the perfect weight." I regret it all.

I'm tired of the ever-changing landscape of information about which foods we should and shouldn't be eating, how to keep our bodies in tip-top shape, how to outsmart the inevitability of aging, the naturalness of cellulite, and the unpredictable possibilities of disease. I'm hoping that you, like a growing number of other women, are tired of hearing about it, too. Trying to eat in a way that defies our natural body types or the aging process is burdensome, futile, misguided, and downright dangerous. Throughout this book, we'll unpack the many ways these unrealistic expectations harm us and our daughters. Not only do we need to question a culture that teaches us that achieving a certain body type and level of physical health is an esteemed and virtuous goal, we also need to acknowledge the ironic and unfortunate fact that a certain harm is caused to each and every one of us who feel the intense and unrelenting pressure to do to it.

In this book, I share something different. I share the healing approach I use to create and embrace a happy, healthy relationship with appetite, body, food, and weight. I use it in my own life, I share it with my daughters, and I also guide countless mothers raising girls to use it.

The positive approach I use to parenting around food is called the Intentional Feeding Mindset (IFM). The IFM centers around **five "touchstones"** that we'll cover in later chapters: **influence, well-being, trust, acceptance, and simple nutrition**. It is at the core of every counseling session, tool, and strategy that I've shared with mothers both in my private practice and through every education, group, program, and workshop I offer via my private practice and NourishHer.com.

The IFM is designed to do three things. First, it inspires you to get curious about any conflicts you're feeling personally and internally with regard to eating, food, and weight, as well as giving you a good reason to resolve them. In doing so, you'll ease the confusion, unsettling discomfort, and tension that can crop up inside you when you're faced with making decisions about what to serve your family, what and how much your kids like to eat and don't eat, and what to eat yourself.

The IFM is also designed to support you externally. If you, like myself and so many of my clients, are finding that conflict over foods, eating habits, and weight are starting to crop up between you and your parenting partner, parents, friends, co-workers, child's school, or even the larger community, then developing your own IFM can provide you with more confidence and clarity in navigating those conversations.

Most importantly, the IFM is designed to help you avoid negative (and sometimes harmful) attitudes, behaviors, and conversations about food, eating, and weight that might be causing stress between you and your daughter. Relying on the IFM will ultimately create more room for acceptance, harmony, and love within your relationship, not only at the table but in other areas of life as well. This book will give you a sense of freedom and peace around foods that you crave for yourself and your daughter.

Specifically, you'll be better able to raise a daughter who has:

- A set of eating skills that help her thrive physically and emotionally

- A sense of resilience, acceptance, and appreciation towards her body regardless of where she falls on the weight spectrum now and throughout life

- An innate ability to tune into her natural feelings of hunger and fullness so that she can eat without having to count calories, restrict foods, or measure portions

- An ability to reach her natural, uniquely-appropriate-for-her body weight without interference from restrictive or pressure-filled diets or eating patterns

- The confidence to eat foods that she enjoys without feeling guilt, shame, remorse, or regret

- An ability to eat with others without worrying about being judged

- The know-how to discern when she is eating (or not eating) for emotional reasons (e.g., anxiety, boredom, excitement, fear, joy, worry) without personal judgment, as well as the awareness to ask for help when she needs it

- A positive relationship with movement and an ability to be active in ways that she enjoys or feel right for her

- A set of self-care skills that bolster protection against the noise of diet culture, including knowing how to navigate images in media, social media, peer pressure, and relationships

You may feel that acknowledging these wants isn't necessary because they are impossible to achieve. Or, if you're the idealistic and hopeful sort, you might think you don't even need to acknowledge them—they should just *be*. And yet these worries still rise up with each snack and meal for almost every parent I have ever worked with in nutrition counseling, including those who haven't ever struggled with eating and dieting themselves.

WHY GIRLS?

While writing this book, people have asked me, *but why girls?*

On my good days, I regard this question as hopeful; perhaps the link between being female and being concerned about the size and shape of your body is not as strong as it once was. Other days, I know the question is a reflection of the sad fact that eating disorders and neurotic worry about foods, eating, and weight is an experience that people of all gender identities can now relate to. The pressure to eat and look a certain way doesn't just impact girls. A growing number of boys, particularly those involved in sports and who fall into racial, ethnic, and sexual minorities are struggling with eating disorders with extra emphasis placed on their muscularity, as opposed to being thinner.[1] In fact, I'd argue that to live in a country that is rife with diet culture, eating elitism, and food disparities means that inevitably *everyone*—regardless of age, gender, race, or sexual identity—is left feeling conflicted, confused, and overly focused on issues related to food, body, and weight.

All that being said and is true, disordered eating and eating disorders are still problems that inordinately impact girls or those who identify as female. Up to three times as many women as men experience three of the most common eating disorders, including anorexia, binge eating disorder, and bulimia.[2] In one longitudinal study, an estimated 51 percent of girls ages 11 to 18 have experienced disordered eating, compared to 34 percent of similarly aged boys.[3] And 75 percent of women of various ages and races reveal that worry about body shape and weight interferes with their happiness.[4] Girls—and the women raising them—deserve particular attention about what it takes to grow up free from diet culture.

Those inequities aside, there's an even simpler reason I'm choosing to focus on girls: Girls are what I know. I was once a girl, I've been a daughter, and I'm now a woman raising girls. I want to speak to you not just as a nutrition professional, but from my own life, my own experiences. I want to start this conversation—and I know that if I do, then women smarter, bolder, and more insightful than I will elevate and continue it by sharing their own experiences.

Of course, I'm not alone. For centuries, issues of worth, identity, and position have played out in the somatic experience of women and girls. If you are raised a woman in America, it's highly likely you have struggled in some way at one time or another in your relationship with your own body. If you are raising another female, it's likely that those conflicts will resurface either as a memory of your own experience or as you witness your daughter wrestle with her own changing body or weight. Inevitably, that struggle will play out in both her and your feelings about food and weight and your attitudes and approach to eating. As mothers and women, we need to break our silence about our own experiences—and we need to better understand those of our daughters. We need to be aware of the issues at play and vigilant in our promise to avoid transmitting our ambivalence to the next generation. If not addressed, an obsession with body and weight threatens to steal the attention of not just our own daughters, but of generations of girls to come.

Lastly, I need to draw attention to the fact that we need other voices in this conversation. We need more stories about foods and eating and the obsession with dieting and weight. We need to hear more stories from women whose experiences are intricately interwoven with other aspects of their identity, including their race, ethnicity, gender identity, socioeconomic class, and personal and cultural values. We all need to speak out together so we can learn to enjoy our bodies and our appetites without judgment and in peace—and to teach the next generation to take this same kind of thinking for granted.

SHALL WE DO THIS?

I invite you to join me in this opportunity to transform your eating life and that of your daughter's. I cherish your company on this journey into what it takes to raise a girl free from worry about her weight and who enjoys eating without fear or regret.

In this book, you'll learn how to develop your own personal Intentional Feeding Mindset (IFM), an approach to feeding you can use to get unstuck from feeding and eating issues that trip you up the most. Together, we will explore evidence-based approaches to feeding as well as explore the deeper feelings that creep up when we try to use them.

By the end of our time together, I hope you will feel like so many of the mothers I have worked with in private nutrition counseling and through NourishHer's workshops and programs. You'll feel a newfound joy in eating and earn the well-deserved ability to feel more *relaxed* about food, meals, feeding your family, and even feeding yourself.

If you're ready to change your inner world at the table as well as put more positive change into the outer world, I'm waiting for you—along with thousands of other moms and their daughters—right here within the pages of this book. Join us!

HOW TO USE THIS BOOK

THROUGHOUT THIS BOOK, YOU WILL FIND THREE TYPES OF RE-sources: **bookmarks, reflections**, and **touchstones**. Each is meant to substantiate information and research-backed concepts, deepen your personal insight, and keep you guided and on track with your increasing ability to build your IFM. Use them if you find them helpful, and feel free to ignore them if you do not. Your ability to support your daughter with her eating will increase substantially, regardless.

BOOKMARKS

 Inspiring and intelligent activists, academics, and fellow registered dietitian nutritionists have written incredible and comprehensive books on important topics covered in this book. Rather than rehash the evidence that they have already covered so adeptly, I want to refer you to those resources and experts themselves directly. The purpose of this book is not to convince you of ideas such as the Satter Eating Competence Model (ecSatter), Health at Every Size® (HAES®), intuitive eating, or weight science by listing multiple bodies of evidence—which can be distracting and confusing—but rather to help you *apply* these concepts to the ways you parent your daughter when it comes to food and eating.

If you want to deepen your knowledge to better apply it to your family or professional practice, or want to help someone else (such as a parenting partner, extended family member, educator, or coach) deepen their own understanding, you will have an excellent set of trustworthy resources to help you dive deeper into specific research-heavy topics to help you do it.

REFLECTIONS

 You are your own best expert in the topic of *you*. You are a unique mix of biology, history, experience, knowledge, beliefs, and values. As a nutrition therapist, I believe it is my job not to *tell* you what to do, but to instead listen to your personal beliefs and goals, then provide you with the relevant information and education that I think will best support you in reaching them. I respect all that you are, all that you know, and all that you have lived. With that in mind, it is only right that I leave it up to *you* to decide if and how you'd like to apply the information I share. Some clients find this liberating and empowering. Some find it scary and challenging. If you're in the second group, not to worry. I won't simply toss out information and expect you to run with it. To help you go deeper into it and how you apply it, I offer you a series of reflective questions at the end of each chapter to support you. Why so many questions? Because leading with curiosity—not advice or criticism—has proven itself over and over again to be the most effective, positive, and powerful ways to help my clients, patients, and myself evolve and grow.

Here are some tips to make the reflection questions more powerful and impactful for you:

- Don't just read the questions. Challenge yourself by taking time to answer them.

- Go slowly. If a question is triggering or challenging, note that with a check mark and move on.

- Take a moment to write down your answers; we know from research that the act of writing itself is therapeutic and healing.[5] If you can't write or simply hate writing, type the answers into a document on your computer or speak them into a note on your phone.

- Use a workbook. To make this easier to do the transformative work, I've put all the questions into one document, which you can download for free at: NourishHer.com/workbook

- Review the questions that were triggering or especially challenging or that you simply wanted to avoid. Typically, the questions that challenge us most are the ones we get the biggest benefit from exploring. If you have a history of food or weight trauma or you're simply not comfortable with or don't feel safe answering certain questions, enlist the help of a mental health professional to support you while you read. To paraphrase the psychoanalyst Carl Jung, what you resist, persists. When we have the courage to face those issues we want to run from most, we will likely make the biggest differences for ourselves and our daughters.

TOUCHSTONES

When you find a Touchstone box, use it as a chance to check in with your own intention regarding your approach to talking to your daughter about food, as well as an opportunity to strengthen your mindset about feeding. If your intention is to protect her from the pain of dieting and weight worry, what is the mindset shift you might need to make based on what you learned in the chapter in order to do so? Taking time to write responses to the **Reflections** can help you get unstuck from old thinking patterns or unhelpful beliefs. Doing so will change both your and your daughter's relationship with food and body in positive, long-lasting ways.

PROLOGUE

THE FIRST TIME I HEARD THE SOUND I WAS STANDING AT THE kitchen sink, giving our breakfast dishes an obligatory rinse before stacking them in the dishwasher. I felt my eight-year-old at my side, whispering an indecipherable question.

"What?" I asked, irritated by her sheepishness, which was a sure sign that she knew her question was one I probably didn't want to hear. Maybe it was to use the iPad "to play Prodigy." To skip soccer "just this one time"? To borrow my phone "for just one teeny second"?

"What?" I pressured louder, my voice charging down at her. Silence. I stopped my cleaning, took a deep breath, and wiped my hands on the closest dish cloth. I noticed her. Her shoulders were rounded and her eyes stared down, in tune with nothing but the grain of the beams of the hardwood floor. The glimpse of the back of her head revealed the messy unraveling of yesterday's braids and reminded me of the time and the fact that I still needed to run a brush through both of my girls' hair.

"Mommy?" she repeated with even less certainty. "Mommy, can I please have another piece of toast?" And there it was, the clear and piercing sound of shame.

No matter how much I'd promised myself I would raise this girl to own her hunger, to love her body, to take joy in her appetite, in that moment her voice spoke the truth. I had failed. Here, my sweet, sensitive daughter was telling me both, "I want this" and also, "I shouldn't want this." That's when I knew I'd need to dig deeper and do more—so much more—if I wanted to make sure her relationship with food would be nothing like mine own.

CHAPTER ONE
EATING WHILE FEMALE

"I do not know why I turned to food. Or do I. I was lonely and scared and food offered an immediate satisfaction. Food offered comfort when I needed to be comforted and did not know how to ask for what I needed from those who loved me. Food tasted good and made me feel better. Food was the one thing within my reach."

—*Roxane Gay, Hunger*

I AM ONE OF THE LUCKY ONES. AND I AM GRATEFUL.
Unlike nearly 30 million other Americans, I've never been diagnosed with an eating disorder. I was never hospitalized—or worse—due to my often odd and sometimes extreme eating (and not eating) behaviors. What I did have was a sort of chronic, almost undetectable pattern of avoiding, controlling, limiting, micromanaging, restricting, researching, obsessing about, and binging on food. Today, as a clinical professional, I can look back on my relationship with food and see that it has been chaotic, disruptive, unbalanced, and even at times downright dangerous. It has certainly been disordered.

Of course, you don't need to be a dietitian to regard my eating behaviors as confusing, disordered, unbalanced, unsound, or plain ol' screwed up. Objectively, *anyone* would question the sanity of a person who regularly chooses to lie in bed with a belly aching with hunger despite being just a few rooms away from a kitchen full of perfectly available, inviting, and nourishing food. Wouldn't they? Similarly, anyone would question my decision to cut out certain macronutrients such as carbs or fat from my diet for days, weeks, even months at a time, wouldn't they? And surely anyone would raise an eyebrow at my insistence on eating only raw foods—nothing heated to above 104 degrees—for months at a time, despite them being painfully difficult to digest and unpleasant to eat.

And, of course, anyone would be concerned by my refusal to eat outside a short four-hour timeframe each day, despite meaning I missed dozens of meals with my family and friends. And my decision to cut out dozens of nutritious foods, including avocado, cauliflower, cabbage, spinach, and peanuts because they weren't considered "right" for me based on my blood type, that would certainly seem strange to anyone. Surely people would question my resolute commitment to doing multiple ten-day-long cleansing "fasts" that included nothing except a mixture of water, maple syrup, lemon, and cayenne pepper. And, of course, people would regard my relentless habit of measuring, weighing, and logging every morsel, filling notebooks upon notebooks, spreadsheets upon spreadsheets, and apps upon apps with numbers after numbers as the sure sign of a problem. Wouldn't they?

Unfortunately, no; they didn't. Instead of being seen as unbalanced, misguided, or pathological, many of my eating behaviors in my teens, twenties, and thirties were accepted, applauded, and encouraged by my mother, family, and friends. In fact, we all referred to it quite innocently as "dieting."

And why *should* anyone have been worried? I always looked well-fed—naturally chubby or plump, never thin—and worked out religiously. Plus, my eating behaviors were the same ones recommended by best-selling authors, celebrities, doctors, journalists, television hosts, and wellness experts of all kinds.

Today, as a nutritionist, I've listened to hundreds of stories about eating and not eating in ways that have nothing to do with appetite or hunger. I've listened to clients, parents, and patients share their stories of limiting and restricting according to dozens of rules that defy common sense and sound science. And for every one of those stories, I've never, ever heard a happy, healthy ending. Instead, with every lengthy restraint from food, there's more often an equal span of binge-ing and repenting.

The chaotic eating patterns I once had aren't just terrifyingly common among my peers or within my practice. One survey of over 4000 women ages 25 to 45 identified that as many as 70 percent of us experience disordered eating—and nearly one-third report spending at least half of our lives since the age of 18 restricting calories.[1] It's not surprising given that popular culture and the medical community sanction restrictive and unbalanced approaches to eating and inextricably intertwine managing our weight as a method to achieving "good health." (More on the multiple ways this is an egregious and ineffective approach later in Chapter 5.) Dieting seems to take a special toll on women. When researchers compared dieting's impact on self-esteem, they found that women experienced a decrease when dieting and focusing on their body shape while men didn't. Men, in fact, experienced increased self-esteem and had fewer body shape concerns when dieting.[2]

Whether you're dieting to lose weight or to be healthy doesn't matter. As you'll learn in this book, eating is meant to be a body-led and joyful experience, not a cognitive and fearful one, nor one that should be driven by a desire to control the size and shape of your body. We do best nutritionally, as well as physically, emotionally, and socially, when we approach eating as the pleasurable, somatic, and necessary daily experience it is meant to be.

Additionally, I believe as women our relationships with food are complicated by much *more* than just a desire to be thinner or live a longer life. Restrained and restrictive ways of eating, regardless of whether their overt goal is weight loss or good health, are often a signal that we feel the need to restrict and restrain ourselves in deeper ways: our ambitions, our creative selves, our desires, and our voices. Rigid and regimented ways of approaching eating are disordered and unhealthy.

And disordered eating (aka dieting) is a precursor to eating disorders, which are catastrophic.

To serve our daughters—and generations of girls to come—we must better understand what is behind the deep and complex connections women make between their sense of selves, their bodies, and food.

WHEN WEIGHT WORRY BEGINS

Like most women, my uneasy relationship with my body started early and it had everything to do with my weight. I remember, for instance, being in first grade and standing in the girls' department of B. Altman looking for a dress for my first communion. A saleswoman took a look at me and directed my mother away from the clothing rack she was thumbing through, toward another where she assured her that she could find something "more appropriate for a big-boned girl." While I felt my mother tense, she took her subtle humiliation in stride and quietly shifted lanes to the nearby rack. A wave of heat still comes over me nearly 40 years later, recalling that moment, the dress we bought, and the tag with the clothing size inside which felt like a scarlet letter, even though only my mother and I could see it.

I also remember a bulletin board in the front of my fourth-grade classroom. It was filled with cardboard milk bottle cutouts. Each bottle stapled to the wall displayed three lines listing a student's name, height, and weight. My stomach tightens when I think of those bottles, the rows and rows, sending out a crisp and clear message to the classroom in their primary colors. The numbers posted there shouted to everyone: *You're the heaviest one in the class!*

My elementary school experience is not unique nor out of date. If you scroll through discussions among women and parents in anti-diet, body-positive, and eating disorder recovery accounts, groups, and hashtags on Facebook and Instagram, you can find similar recounts of being called out in school among peers because of weight—albeit in more direct and humiliating ways. Even today, my own daughters' schools each ask for their Body Mass Index (BMI) measurement at the start of the school year. Across the country, many states still require schools to measure and assess children's BMI and, in some cases, flag the status of kids in larger bodies to parents. This is done despite the fact that there's a lack of research or consensus on the benefits of this focus on BMI; furthermore, multiple research studies indicate there are significant and negative impacts of focusing on a child's weight.[3]

Regardless of whether a school puts extra emphasis on a child's BMI, it's not unusual for young girls to be concerned about their weight. Researchers have documented that 81 percent of ten-year-old girls reported they were afraid of being fat; 42 percent of first-through-third graders say they want to be thinner; 51 percent of nine- and 10-year-old girls reported that they were "sometimes" or "very often" on diets, and 82 percent of their families were "sometimes" or "very often" on diets.

Pre-adolescent and early adolescent girls are primed to focus on their body shape and size, thanks to a host of factors that converge during these years. Developmentally, it's a time when peer acceptance is important and children want to be as similar to friends of the same age as possible. It's also a time when binary thinking is still common: you're either "thin" or "fat," which, thanks to the culture we live in, also often happens to equate to right and wrong, good and bad, with little room for anything in between. And as girls are approaching and transitioning into puberty, their body shape changes rapidly, including increases in fat stores. This perfectly healthy and normal change can feel out of control and uncomfortable in a fat-phobic world. Dieting might seem like a cure to avoid that discomfort.

"With early adolescence, girls surrender their relaxed attitudes about their bodies and burden themselves with self-criticism," says Mary Pipher, PhD, in her book *Reviving Ophelia: Saving the Selves of Adolescent Girls*. Adolescence is a time when a girl is most at risk of turning away from her authentic self in favor of creating what Alice Miller calls a "false self," which is a self that favors meeting societal expectations and cultural ideals. It's a time when Simone deBeauvoir says girls go from "being to seeming." It's the time when we watch our girls go from natural, relaxed, comfortable, and uninhibited to self-conscious, insecure, tense, and unsure. And it's not surprising that this struggle is at least partially played out in the body.

As I write this, I'm thinking of my own daughter, who at nine skips unabashedly down the sidewalk in front of me, braids swinging, as we walk into town. She seems to be trying with each skip to see if she can pull her knee up higher. It never occurs to her to wonder how her body looks to the rest of the world, only how she can feel and make it move. She's a beautiful contrast to the two middle school girls on the other side of the street, wearing a uniform of high cut denim shorts and flannel shirts tied in knots at the waist, long hair blown straight, who are giggling towards one another shyly and doing little else but seeming to hope to be seen.

Notably, it's also a time when mothers can have a significant impact on their daughters' perception of themselves. Pipher goes on to say that adolescence is a time "when gender roles get set in cement, and that's when girls need tremendous support in resisting the cultural definitions of femininity." The key for mothers, I believe, is being aware of the deeper drama that is going on inside our adolescent daughters when we see them wage war on their bodies by dieting. It's to understand that their struggle with their body is not truly about being "thin," "healthy," or "fit;" it's a struggle with identity, personal power, place in the world, and self-worth. Our desire to help our daughters remain in touch with their authentic selves—the selves who can skip down the street and focus on what they *are* instead of how they look—isn't just admirable, it's imperative. To succeed, we as mothers and role models can help by acknowledging our own histories with and feelings about our bodies, food, eating, and our understanding of weight.

WHEN WEIGHT WORRY ESCALATES

While I was aware, critical, and self-conscious of my body in grade school, I didn't actively start trying to change it until middle school. My body was starting to swell with the changes of puberty and it seemed to be making me—and what felt like all the adults around me, including my mother—extremely uneasy. Dieting seemed like a way to escape from the uninvited force that was shape-shifting me from girl to woman, as well the pressures and new identity that seemed to be coming along with those changes. By the time I was in ninth grade, a strange tension around food overwhelmed me. Controlling the urge to eat felt like a way to control everything else that made me so ill at ease with myself. I remember being in the high school cafeteria, eating baked potatoes and mustard with an occasional side of pretzels before soccer. That's sacrilege by today's low-carb dieting standards; back then it was fat grams that terrorized those of us who dreamed of being skinny.

Dieting for me, like so many others, proved to be a slippery slope. When counting grams wasn't quite as effective as I'd hoped it would be, I took matters into my own hands. At some point in high school, I got hip to the idea of purging. I'm not sure where I heard about it—a teen magazine, a friend? Vomiting and laxatives were an outlet for my obsessive longing to be less fleshy. I was desperate to erase the swelling of my hips, minimize the widening of my thighs, and cure whatever else was making me feel so ill at ease in myself. While I loathed and was humiliated by it—the private visits to the bathroom, the mess, the hiding sounds and smells—I kept working at it anyway. And if my mother or friends ever suspected it, no one mentioned it. It made sense that my awkward exits after meals went unaddressed; in those days, an eating disorder required an emaciated body. Visually speaking, in my case there appeared very little to worry about. While I'd complain constantly about my body, how big I felt, and how fat I looked, my weight remained unchanged and to everyone I appeared "healthy," if not still in need of losing a few pounds by idealized standards.

When I think back on those years, I feel a range of emotions—shame, bewilderment, anger, to name a few—but mostly I am amazed by my luck. By the grace of some unknown force, I gave up my purging behaviors around the time I graduated high school. Instead of celebrating wildly about the fact that I escaped a full-on eating disorder, I berated myself for not having what I thought of as the will and strength of other girls who could grit it out through this particular type of pain, torture, and self-destruction. While I finished my senior year and went off to NYU with my fat fully intact, the girls I'd passed by in those school bathrooms, the girls I envied, were missing several semesters of college and suffering other losses that I can only now imagine were much worse.

Despite that triumphant failure, throughout my twenties, my thoughts, hopes, and dreams all continued to revolve around achieving an admirable level of svelteness. I was always on a diet or off a diet. I was either forcibly trying to push my weight down or shamefully letting it creep back up. Every form of movement I engaged in was dominated by an aggressive attempt at tightening, toning, and reshaping. Restricting and eliminating. Berating and hating. They dominated my life over and over and over. Whenever I was successful at being smaller, the compliments and encouragement I'd get from everyone around me would push me to pursue dieting's redemptive promises with even more tenacity.

Over the years, I gained weight and lost it. Gained and lost. Gained and lost. My obsession gnawed at my self-esteem, stole me away from what would have otherwise been happy moments, and battle-axed any unrelated ambition. While undetectable to others, it occupied my mind at every meal, with every bout of hunger or mention of food, with every significant holiday or event, with every purchase of clothing, and with every photograph. Season after season it tortured me. If you ask me about any significant moment in my life, I can likely recall my exact body weight at the time. A number on a bathroom scale defined me— like so many other women I have known—in a way that nothing else seemed to.

Not surprisingly, my obsession dominated not just my personal life but also my career. It was the fuel that helped me land coveted positions at different women's magazines. I poured all my creative energy and dieting acumen into researching and writing stories about fitness, nutrition, and weight loss and tried to help other women lose weight too. I did my best to fulfill the wants of the senior editors above me who, in what I can only imagine was an effort to keep their own jobs, constantly requested we produce features about enviable weight-loss successes, celebrity secrets for staying slim, and workouts that promised to correct all manner of femininity's physical shortcomings. Collectively, we stoked the fires of dieting's empty promises for the billions of women just like me who believed them.

THE GOOD FORTUNE OF FAILING

When it came to actively restricting food, I felt little shame. Dieting, as it turns out, is a great connector, a social bridge, and a matter of pride. I had no problem sharing the obscure food rules I was following with other women I knew. Of course, while I allowed the limiting aspects of my pursuits to be wholly visible, I made sure that the darker side of my dieting—the rebound eating and eating and eating—was not. I considered the rebound eating and weight gain to be clear evidence that I was a total and complete failure.

As the years and years of dieting went on, my inner eater became much stronger than my restricting self. Several days into any new well-planned eating regimen, a rebel in me would rise up. My restraint would unravel. The holding back, the constriction, the subversion of my hunger and my appetite would explode into fits of binges on butter cookies, jars of Nutella, containers of frosting, cartons of ice cream, and anything else sickeningly sweet that I could get my hands on. Bingeing after a day or two of dieting was always an orgasmic release. It felt as if my inner wanting was bursting out of that self-inflicted prison. In those moments, eating with abandon seemed a violent act against authority, against beauty, against fitting in, against perfection and a host of other invisible forces that I felt were repressing me. I was angry, and the eating and overeating gave me sweet relief. Though I didn't regard it as such at the time, the fact that my hunger would win out over my will to subvert my wanting was a miraculous triumph. My appetite was an unlikely savior.

Looking back now, I see my binges as my deepest self, rising up from within. My will to eat and eat was an undeniable signal of something buried that begged to push through the surface. Unfortunately, it'd be years before I'd allow it to happen. After every binge I'd confront my still-not-perfect body in the mirror. As I scrutinized my own image, my insecurities and self-loathing would well up again. That hungry rebel in me would die and I would turn back to dieting, limiting, and restricting food and denying my hunger all over again.

Here's the good news: at some point in my early thirties, I experienced a merciful turning point. It came in the form of time and space with myself. For the first time in my life, I was alone. My social life quieted. My closest friends—women whom I'd known since middle school and college—were distracted by their careers, marriages, and growing families. In a moment of courage, I quit my staff job in an editorial office and decided to become a freelancer. I bought a small studio apartment in a town where I knew no one. I was lonely, and in that loneliness, my chaotic, chasing, and obsessive mind started to relax. In the quiet, my body and its true hunger and rhythms became known to me. Through a messy mix of maturity, education, self-help books, introspection, and fatigue, I started to see my eating issues for what they were: a huge distraction from myself. I rediscovered books that I'd been drawn to, collected, and moved in boxes from apartment to apartment over the years. Books I had always been too broken or distracted or starving to read or understand and yet never quite ready to part with. Through writings by Kim Chernin, Alice Miller, Mary Pipher, Evelyn Tribole, and others, my curiosity about my battle with my body began to grow. (You will hear my favorite insights from these daring and beautiful souls throughout this book.) Through them, I made three discoveries that triggered a powerful shift in my relationship with eating and dieting. If you are struggling, I'm confident they'll help set you, too, free from dieting's allure and empty promises.

ACCEPTING MY HUNGER

First, I confronted a truth: Dieting is futile. I found my own proof of this fact when my mother moved out of our childhood home. While cleaning out boxes and books from my bedroom, I was confronted with years of handwritten records of my dieting. They were scribbled on jagged pieces of scrap paper and stashed inside recipe books, neatly written inside leather-bound journals, quickly jotted down on the backs of notebooks, noted in the margins of recipes, written on an index card preserved inside a Ziploc bag, typed up in emails and in Excel spreadsheets, then printed and stowed in manila folders. There were logs of calories, fat grams, carb counts, exercise reps, glasses of water, minutes, miles, pounds, body fat percentages, and breast, waist, hip, thigh, and calf measurements. And in those numbers was undeniable evidence. According to the logs, my body weight would trend up as soon as I set my mind to losing it. First, I would drop a pound, or two, or ten, then the numbers would start rising back up, then the records would stop for a few weeks or months, only to start back up again. Since my freshman year in high school—over twenty years of dieting, gaining and losing, painfully hating and denying—I had a net change of four pounds.

By the time I became a dietitian, I'd discovered that my weight loss failures were a biological mechanism designed to protect me. My body had an optimal weight, and no matter what nutritional torture and deprivation I put it through, it was resilient and powerful in its ability to maintain it. By the time I started unearthing research studies indicating the same, I was primed and ready to believe them. Despite what diet and health culture had trained me to believe, my body did not want to be smaller. My body was, in fact, diet-proof, and if I wanted to live a full life undistracted and unharmed, then it was time to start embracing it.

The second discovery that helped set me free from dieting was this: My instinct to eat and eat and eat whenever I felt restricted wasn't a nuisance—it was a rebel voice from within. In time, I learned to listen to it. I started to understand that my bingeing wasn't a failure, a lack of willpower, a shameful form of gluttony, or a sign of unruly hedonism. It was a heroine that refused to let me ignore my hunger, subvert my pleasure, or deny my appetite. When I denied my hunger by dieting, my bingeing would surface as a powerful reminder that I did not want to be hungry and numb, I wanted to be fed and live.

My eating—and overeating—was just as much a response to the starving I was doing as it was to the uncomfortable, confusing emotions I was feeling, not just about my body but my place in the world. Since that time, I've come to regard those days when I feel compelled to eat and eat and eat as a great sign that something inside me needs to be heard and it is either too fearful or unsure to come through. I now know that an overwhelming or insatiable appetite is my body speaking to me—and I need to feed it as a form of self-care, be it with food or rest or movement or other. And, more importantly, I need to make time to breathe deep, get quiet, and listen.

Finally, I unearthed an unpopular realization: My weight did not need to matter as much as I'd been trained to believe, not to my health at least. My disordered eating habits, my restricting and overeating, my weight cycling, my irregular and extreme exercise regimens, were more harmful than helpful. As it turns out, yo-yoing isn't just mentally exhausting; it's physically taxing on the heart and metabolic and hormonal systems. And if my body weight was best left to fall where it may, the only thing left was to work on accepting it. For several years after I made those discoveries, I gradually started to eat and move in ways that were more ordered than disordered and that made me more happy than unhappy. I felt more at peace with and grateful for my body.

Bookmark: *What We Don't Talk About When We Talk About Fat* by Aubrey Gordon. My own struggles with my body and weight have felt very real powerful and real to me; however, thanks to the work of Gordon, I've come to be able to see my experience as part of a larger context of what other people in other bodies across the weight spectrum endure. I now know my body's relative proximity to the thin ideal has protected me outwardly from the significant harms of anti-fat bias. If you or your daughter (teenage or older) would like to understand fatness as a social justice issue, this book and Gordon's podcast Maintenance Phase are excellent places to start.

DANCING ON THE EDGE

My journey away from dieting has not been linear. It has been a gradual awakening, a circling in and out of obsession and clarity. It's been three steps forward with understanding and peace, then two steps back with every situation of stress or change in body—marriage, pregnancy, motherhood, aging. Fantasies about how toning up, slimming down, running, spinning, lifting, and cleaning up my eating will fix everything return. Then I remember that they are lies.

I'm sharing my story because it's far from unique. The journey that sends a woman into war with her body begins early—by some reports, as young as six years old.[2] By the time they reach college age, 91 percent of women report having been on at least one diet.[4]

Millions of women have a story that is less extreme than mine, and millions of others have stories that are more intense, painful, and disruptive. For those of us who are lucky enough to be able to say we are no longer actively engaged in battle with every meal and every pound gained or lost, there is still a risk that old habits and attitudes are alive just beneath the surface. Despite our best intentions, the idea that cleaning up our eating can earn us our redemption is constantly reinforced by culture, by the medical community, by pseudo-experts and celebrities, and by all-pervasive social media. It's a full-time job to have a healthy defense against the pressure to diet and diet culture, a culture that brilliant activist and dietitian Christy Harrison, MPH, RD, aptly refers to as the "Life Thief" in her groundbreaking and comprehensive book on the subject, *Anti-Diet: Reclaim Your Time, Money, Well-Being, and Happiness Through Intuitive Eating*. It's not until we drum up the courage to face our deepest issues with eating and not eating and overeating and weight—what I call our "food 'ish"—that we can break the destructive cycles we spin in.

When we become mothers (and teachers, caregivers, mentors, and role models to girls), guarding against the pervasive pressure of diet culture becomes infinitely more important. We are so vital to helping our daughters accept the natural shape and size of their body because we are the ones who pass on the notion of what it means to be a woman. If we are intentional, we can resist the inclination to pass on traditional ideals. Instead, we can encourage our daughters to remain true to their authentic selves, including their appetites, their bodies, and their appearance.

To understand now, as a parent and a healthcare professional, what a delicate line I teetered between dieting and full-blown eating disorder (ED), is terrifying. While I danced wildly on that precipice, constantly in danger of descending into a full-blown ED, I never quite slipped or tripped off the ledge. It'd be empowering to think it was my inner self that held back, that didn't collapse into madness completely. To understand the pathology of eating disorders is to know that it was not my inner reserve—it was simple luck. For whatever reasons, some of us don't have that specific trifecta of environment, genetics, and personality type that researchers are coming to understand is at the heart of the most deadly and perpetuating forms of eating disorders. And for whatever reasons, some of us do. It's impossible to know who can sway on the edge of dieting without falling to a depth that's tragically and notoriously (often impossibly) difficult to battle back from. With that in mind, it's important to demand that our daughters never dance there to begin with.

HOW MOTHERS FIT IN

If my mother had known what we as mothers know now, if she had been aware of the fact that dieting was a type of disordered eating, a risk factor for a full-blown eating disorder, linked with increased weight gain and lowered self-esteem, and a trigger that could worsen anxiety or depression, I'd like to think she would have intervened in a different sort of way. But she didn't.

In the late 80s in our suburban town just north of New York City, being successful at dieting—not the risk of dieting—was the topic of conversations, magazine articles, and television shows. The fact that my mother regularly made time to head to Weight Watchers meetings in the evenings after a full day at the office, cooked full dinners for myself and my brother and then opted for something smaller and "lighter" on her own plate, or pushed herself to do rounds of sit-ups and jumping jacks in front of the television at night seemed normal, if not noble. In my eyes, my mother's detailed attention to her appearance, the amount of time and effort she put into looking in the mirror to ensure her clothing lay just right, and the effort she put into trying to be slim seemed to be part of her strength. As a young woman, I never thought to question it. In fact, when she allowed me to join her in it, I was flattered.

If my mother had seen my discomfort with my body and my weight as I see it today, I like to think she'd have done things differently. If she had seen my wanting to lose weight as a symptom of those deeper struggles that occur during adolescence—such as changing identity, social stress, depression, anxiety, and questioning my place in the world—then perhaps she wouldn't have intervened by helping me stay small, but instead encouraged me to fight against that urge. Maybe she would have also taken steps to protect me from her own issues with keeping up appearances and provided me with other avenues for boosting esteem and feelings of power instead. If she had had the pieces of information that mothers of girls are striving to hear now, the next two decades of my life back then likely would have belonged to me—not to my relentless obsession with my weight.

Instead, I think my mother did what so many other mothers still feel forced to do. She danced between the devil and the deep blue sea. She felt the cultural pressure to be thin and she also resented it. She worried about my increasing weight—the harm a larger body might cause me socially—and wanted to support me when she saw me worrying about it. And yet she worried about my dieting, too. There was a great contradiction that seeped into every meal, every decision about dessert, and every confrontation with a clothing store mirror. It was, "Have more, you hardly had anything," alongside, "If you eat that you'll be sorry, it's loaded with calories!" And, "Oh my gosh, stop complaining, you look great," moments before, "Don't worry; you always lose it fast when you want to." She was caught between wanting to protect me both from developing a body I loathed as much as she did her own and also the guilt I'd feel after eating a full plate of food.

In my practice, I meet so many mothers who are doing this delicate dance themselves with their own daughters. They come to me and say, "She is so unhappy at this weight; please tell her that she shouldn't be eating these things." And in the same session say, "I just want her to be happy with herself; I want her to have a healthy relationship with food and not suffer like I did." Their ambivalence is palpable.

In all truthfulness, I feel for them. I am standing right there with them. While intellectually, I know it's harmful to put so much value on the way a body looks, I, too, get triggered with worry and concern for my daughters when I see them putting on weight or eating in ways that seem terribly "unhealthy" or beyond what I think they should want or need. Just because I can acknowledge the stupidity and harm of misplacing value on body size and looks or catastrophizing every sugary treat into a potential for unhealthy demise, I'd be lying if I said that that knowledge alone was enough to erase the pressure to conform to standards of beauty, "clean eating," or thinness from my mind or life. Yes, some of us will encounter one significant touchpoint—a well-written book, a powerful talk, or the content of a brilliant and radical social justice activist—to change our perspective, but many of us will need more. We will stand in the in-between, both knowing we don't want our daughters to embrace those values and also building up the resilience within ourselves to reject them.

Of course, it's okay to take positive action even if you're in the in-between. I believe it is possible to both acknowledge and understand the harmful nature of diet culture, to be firm in your desire to protect your children from it, and to continue to feel pressured by its unrelenting gaze. You can rage against your phone every time you see a Facebook ad or influencer push a fat-erasing cleanse or detox diet and still grapple with feeling comfortable with how you (or your daughter) looks in a bathing suit. Ambivalence in this arena makes total sense to me. If you still struggle with walking the walk despite believing the anti-diet talk, I am right there with you. We are rallying against a belief system that we have been enveloped in for as long as we have been alive—generations before us, too. Have grace with yourself if there is sometimes doubt and if it doesn't always come easy. And know this for sure: We can take a firm stance that body weight, shape, and size are no measure of self-worth, and we can teach our children how to be joyful, happy, healthy eaters even if we are still working on strengthening those beliefs and our own relationship with food and our bodies ourselves. We must, in fact. If we wait until we are 100 percent there ourselves, there's a chance it will be too late.

STOPPING THE CYCLE

This book is a game plan for anyone like me. It's for the mothers I meet in my practice who want something better for their daughters, who struggle to find that fine line between supporting their daughter's desire to pursue good health and protecting them against the dangers of fixating on the size and shape of their bodies. This book is also for mothers like me who have struggled to overcome an unhealthy relationship with food and eating and want nothing more than to make sure their daughters grow to have a natural ease around food and feel good about their body and weight. This book is filled with tips on managing food, eating, and feeding your family with awareness, confidence, and love.

To build your awareness, this book will illuminate the ways we can get tripped up when we see our daughters struggling with their weight or feelings about eating and food. Through our awareness, we begin to understand that to cheer our daughters on in their effort to reduce their size because it's "what she wants," because it's "normal for girls to worry about their weight," or because a pediatrician has deemed her BMI too high can have unintended and long-term consequences on her self-esteem, eating habits, eating disorder risk, and an increase in body weight.

Our increasing awareness will also help us recognize that a desire to change our body can signal a deeper struggle. We will begin to understand that seeing a daughter reject or lose confidence in her body because of her weight is a sign that she is losing confidence in her self-worth. As Pipher teaches, while we must acknowledge and show empathy for the cultural pressure that can put us at war with our bodies, as mothers we must remain firm that in our value system, her self-worth has absolutely nothing to do with looks or her weight.

We will learn to recognize that when we see our daughters wanting to battle against their bodies, it is our job to step in and help them understand that what they are truly battling is discomfort with themselves and their place in the world. When we wage war against our bodies, we are often attempting to fix a problem with our relationships, lack of power, or worth. When the urge to diet, binge, or reject the natural size and shape of the body arises in our daughters, we will have the awareness to know that the way we can help her most is by avoiding the urge to support her desire to work on or focus on slimming down or toning up and instead, dig deeper into what really ails her.

Throughout this book, I will share what I have learned by listening to adolescent girls who come to me asking for help losing weight. Probing deeper into their ambitions (an exercise you can use yourself and will find later in this book) has revealed valuable insights. Underneath the desire to shed pounds or flatten a tummy or to fit into a prom dress are wants such as, "to feel more comfortable with friends," "to be accepted when I get to college," "to make my parents happy," or "to help me feel more confident." These are the goals that really matter to our girls. Focusing on weight at the expense of overlooking what is really at the core of our daughter's deepest desires is a grave distraction.. Awareness can help us avoid it.

To build your confidence in knowing how best to approach feeding your daughter and talking to her about body, food, and weight, I've identified five touchstones—**influence, well-being, trust, acceptance,** and **simple nutrition**—which collectively I call the **Intentional Feeding Mindset (IFM)**. These touchstones incorporate specific, evidence-based tactics that I teach mothers to use to raise healthy, competent eaters. Once you understand these touchstones, they will be yours to use again and again to steady yourself as challenging issues come up. As your confidence in your stance builds, you'll feel empowered to guide your daughter on a grounded path to comfort, freedom, and acceptance with her decisions about eating, foods, health, and weight. You'll be able to navigate conflict as it arises in yourself, in your relationship with your daughter around foods and weight, and even in larger communities if you feel compelled.

Throughout this book, you will also have an opportunity to build your love. However, this increasing love won't just be for your daughter. Just by picking up this book, you've already proven you hold tremendous love for a young girl in your life. Exercises at the end of each chapter will support you in deepening your love and self-compassion for *yourself* as well. By being curious about your own history, you will better understand the motives, attitudes, and ambivalence about eating, dieting, health, and weight that drive you. By building empathy, compassion, patience, and understanding with yourself, you will model for your daughter the greatest kind of love, which is directed at the self. By drawing on your own experiences, you will carve out the best path forward for yourself and your daughter—one that helps you both grow into more fulfilled versions of yourselves, along with any younger girls you may care for, influence, or meet.

REFLECTIONS ON YOUR HISTORY WITH FOOD

- *Think back to your own childhood. Were mealtimes something that you looked forward to—or were they a source of stress, something you either feared, or wanted to avoid?*

- *As a child, were there rules about which foods you had to eat? How about how much or how little you had to eat? Or would you say that those decisions were left up to you?*

- *Did you feel you had enough food—or do you remember feeling as though you wanted more?*

- *Was there a routine to your meals? Did they usually occur in the same place, with the same people, and at roughly the same times? Or were they more erratic?*

- *Did you diet as a child or young adult? Did your mother, father, or other adult family members diet?*

- *Did your mother, father, or other adult family members comment on your body? Did they comment on your weight?*

- *As a child, did you feel good about your eating? Why or why not?*

To get a complete set of questions,
download the *Diet-Proof* journal at NourishHer.com/workbook.

CHAPTER TWO
CREATING YOUR INTENTIONAL FEEDING MINDSET (IFM)

"My doctor told me I would never walk again. My mother told me I would. I believed my mother."

—*Wilma Rudolph, first American woman to win three Olympic gold medals*

WHAT DO YOU WANT FOR YOUR DAUGHTER?

IF YOU CAME TO SEE ME FOR NUTRITION THERAPY, THERE'S A very good chance I'd start our first session by asking you this question: "What do you want for your daughter—what is your goal?" Sometimes this question catches people off guard. Sometimes, it's followed by several seconds of awkward silence during which I see parents' cheeks flush red or a smidgen of irritation or skepticism cross through their eyes. I assume they're thinking, *You are the expert; shouldn't you be telling me the goal?* In fact, I don't always need to assume. Parents have answered, "I don't know. Why don't *you* tell me?"

Of course, as a nutrition therapist and a co-conspirator on your journey towards the wellness you seek for you and your family, my goal isn't to challenge you. It's to empower you. By giving you a chance to think about what you want for your daughter, I am telling you that your perspective matters. In fact, it matters most.

As a mother, you are one of the singular, most powerful resources your daughter has in the world; your influence is profound. Whether done consciously or not, you're impacting your daughter's sense of self, her values, and what she chooses to prioritize in her own life each and every day. Your influence on her starts from the moment she is born, even before, and will last long after you are gone. This thought is not to scare you, or fill you with pressure or dread. It is to merely call in the truth and give you a moment to choose. It is to help you choose consciously and with intention. While other influences will come and go, yours will remain. I'm nudging you here; be aware of this fact And mostly, be careful not to give your power away—not to her pediatrician, nor parenting experts, nor her therapist, nor teachers, media, culture, and certainly not the most recent best-selling author. Remember that as her mother, you are at the helm—*you*.

I have learned so much from the responses of the mothers I work with. In hundreds of conversations, I've shined a floodlight on where both our confidence and unsureness as mothers most often lie. You see, I believe that when a mother comes to me for help getting her daughter to *eat* better, what she's really asking me is to help her daughter *feel* better. Buried at the heart of every parent's request for my guidance on how to help their child eat more vegetables, lose or gain weight, balance her blood sugar, or stop snacking so much is almost always the same desire. At the heart of every reason a mother makes an appointment to see a doctor, a nutritionist, or therapist or decides to pick up a parenting self-help book is this: **a wish for her daughter to be well**.

Our definition of being well or well-being may differ from mother to mother, parent to parent, and person to person. (More on how to clarify your own defining elements of well-being in Chapter 3). Once we identify our deepest goal for our daughters, then we can anchor ourselves to that intention. The intention acts as a north star, guiding us through even the most challenging decisions we face when it comes to helping our daughters navigate issues related to eating, foods, physical activity, and weight.

You see, eating, feeding, and nutrition are nebulous things. There's no one answer, no one approach, no one right food or diet or nutrient array or intake that is right for every parent or child or person. When you identify your deepest intention for your daughter, it makes it easier to stay the course of your own choosing when it comes to deciding which eating, food, and food decisions are right for you—and more importantly, for her. You'll be protected from being hoodwinked, sidetracked, or distracted by every new eating trend, well-meaning friend or family member who shares their own advice, or the latest dieting best-seller or food-or-exercise claim that comes into view. When faced with alternative advice, views, and recommendations, you can run them through your very own truth-o-meter. Does this align with my goal for my daughter? Will this bring her closer to that goal—or will this widen the gap more? As you work deeper in this book, you'll have even more specific questions to ask as a protection against dieting, diet culture, and harm to your deepest goals for your daughter. Those questions will align with building trust and acceptance, and increasing enjoyment and well-being.

For mothers with a history of dieting, we can bolster protection against uncomfortable feelings about food (and the pleasure we get from it), physical activity (and the punitive, obligatory attitudes we have towards it), and body weight (and the bias and judgment we internalize about it) by going a step further and aligning ourselves with a very specific tool I've developed, and which you can make your own, using the exercises in this book. It is called the *Intentional Feeding Mindset*.

WHAT IS THE INTENTIONAL FEEDING MINDSET (IFM)?

The IFM is a practice you'll employ every time you make a decision about what and how much to feed your daughter, as well as what and how much to say about eating, nutrition, and body weight. Using the IFM ensures that your decisions around foods and eating are aligned with your goals for your daughter, your family, and yourself. In time, using the IFM will become automatic, intuitive, and natural.

Investing time in developing your own IFM upfront will help you navigate tricky issues as they come up in day-to-day situations, as well as throughout developmental stages such as elementary school, adolescence, teenage years, and beyond. A solid IFM will ultimately reduce stress during meals and snacks, boost your daughter's self-esteem and, ultimately, strengthen your relationship with your daughter as she will trust that you are operating with consistency from a place of acceptance, confidence, love, and trust.

Developing an IFM isn't about being a perfect feeder or parent; instead, it's an opportunity to get clear on your goals. The IFM gives you the courage to stand by those goals even when outside influences—such as other family members, your daughter's friends, well-meaning (but unaware) doctors, and social media—pressure you to veer away from them.

The IFM also gives you clarity and insight to deal with your own history and feelings about eating, dieting, foods, and weight when they start to surface and threaten to run amuck. Developing your own IFM will help you feel more confident in the daily choices you make around foods and eating, so much so that eventually you will rarely think about them at all. Your self-assurance and ease around foods will transmit to your daughter, creating a solid foundation for her relationship with food and eating that will last throughout her life.

The IFM is based in a framework that comprises five touchstones. From within these touchstones, a healthy, balanced, and joyful approach to eating, foods, physical activity, and weight can grow. Similarly, when a parent is struggling with their child over issues related to foods and eating, reflecting on the touchstones has been an effective way to identify what's at the deeper core of the problem. They can both strengthen your approach and also help highlight sources of weakness. The five touchstones include:

Influence. Regardless of the strength of your intentions for your daughter and yourself, developing a strong IFM requires identifying the many influences that impact your daughter's relationship with food and her thoughts and feelings about her eating, her body, and her weight. This book will provide tips for proactively working against influences that may damage your daughter's self-esteem, such as cultural influences, peers, developmental stages, the medical community, school assignments, social media, and well-meaning family members (including other caregivers). It will also help us recognize the surprising ways our own attitudes towards health and approach to eating might impact our daughters' relationships to food and body.

Well-being. True health is not merely the absence of disease, but rather a state of total emotional, social, and physical well-being. To raise a truly healthy daughter, we must avoid a tendency to overemphasize one area of health at the expense of another. Will we discuss how a focus on eating well-being—eating in a way that supports us emotionally and socially, as well as nutritionally—opposed to traditional notions of healthy eating—which imply eating to support physical health above all else. This can help you make day-to-day eating and feeding decisions that support your daughter holistically, as well as when serious situations come up, such as a diet-related medical diagnoses like diabetes, celiac, or a food allergy or intolerance.

Trust. The more you learn to trust your child's natural instincts around foods and eating, the better your child will be able to trust herself. Just like learning any new skill, we can create an environment that offers both structure and a freedom to make mistakes and learn from them. This book will provide evidence-based tools that can help you trust your daughter to learn to have a satisfying, enjoyable, and physically nourishing relationship with food, including her eating habits, her appetites, and her hunger. Additionally, you'll also learn about tools and strategies you can use to support her in cultivating a trusting relationship with her body as it is now and with changes that will occur naturally over time, such as through puberty, pregnancy, menopause, aging, physical illness, and emotional or social stress.

Acceptance. Developing your IFM will ask you to see your daughter for who she truly is and encourage you to offer her a precious gift—her own self-acceptance. In order to help your daughter thrive, we will discuss what true acceptance is, how it impacts our feelings about foods, eating, our body, and our well-being as well as what we can do to cultivate and strengthen it. Furthermore, we will be called on to reflect on how we can benefit by being more accepting of our own appetite, food preferences, eating habits, body shape and size, and health status.

Simple Nutrition. You do not need a PhD in nutrition nor the discipline to stick to a regimented eating style in order to raise a great eater. Clinical experience, research, and the tools and strategies shared in this book prove just the opposite, providing you with an essential understanding of the fundamental components of eating well-being. You'll learn how and when to add in special nutrition concerns and food groups—and when and why there are times when you'll do best to avoid them. Ultimately, you'll deepen your understanding of how creating consistency and structure with meals—as opposed to squarely focusing on increasing the number of vegetables you or your daughter eats on any given day—is the very best way to improve nutritional health. It also can ease common eating frustrations, such as food fights and mealtime conflicts, selective eating or picky eating (despite already showing the capacity to enjoy a variety of flavors and textures), an unwillingness to try new or unfamiliar foods, or an inability to eat portion sizes that help maintain a natural, uniquely-appropriate-for-them (not idealized) body weight.

The five touchstones are born out of my own experience working with women, particularly parents of my clients. The touchstones are the areas that I find former dieters tend to get tripped up by the most. For example, one mother I worked with came to me because her daughter's BMI had increased over the past year. She told me repeatedly, "I just want my daughter to have a healthy relationship with food." While I admired the clarity of her desire and gave her my rapt attention, it took me only a few minutes of listening to understand the problem.

Everything this mom shared about a recent weekend with the grandparents was in direct contradiction to her original statement.

"My father always keeps ice cream in the freezer. He doesn't understand that my daughter just can't control herself around those kinds of foods," she shared. "I just want her to understand what's healthy and what isn't. I avoid keeping sugary foods in our apartment because I know they're bad for her, not to mention how they can cause bloating."

On weekend visits, mom had discovered that her daughter had been sneaking and bingeing on the many "forbidden foods" her father kept in his kitchen. While mom was doing her very best to keep her daughter healthy by making the treats she enjoyed off-limits and keeping them out of their home, she inadvertently set her up for feeling out of control around them when given the opportunity to indulge. Conversations about *trust* with food were the starting place for this family.

Consider, also, a sixteen-year-old client who comes to see me for help with weight loss. She's always been in a higher BMI category and has also always been healthy, athletic, and a balanced eater. Mom supports her daughter's weight loss wishes, adding that "all her friends are slimmer, so I totally understand" and she hates "to see her so unhappy." Mom is so blinded by identifying with her daughter's desire to be thin that she fails to see that supporting her sends her the message that she agrees that her body is imperfect as is. By helping her look for a way to lose weight, she's telling her, yes, she'd be better off if she was thinner. There's no eating plan or diet in the world that would cure the food conflicts that were going on between the two of them. At the core of this problem was a hyper-focus on social life (and the risk of her emotions and risk for an eating disorder). Getting in a positive place with food and nutrition and weight was a matter of having a better understanding of the concepts of *well-being* and *acceptance*.

RAISING COMPETENT EATERS

Here is the sweet truth: Mothers who have a structured yet relaxed approach to feeding their daughters raise happier, healthier eaters. To raise a really great eater, you do not need to research and worry about which foods are "bad" and "good," govern over every food your child puts in her mouth, micromanage sweets, or try to discern whether every portion served and eaten is too much or too little. You do not need to be able to give a dissertation on good nutrition nor feel that your child's weight—be it higher or lower than you or your child's pediatrician believes ideal—is your fault or responsibility to change. In fact, taking on that level of responsibility, overseeing too many aspects of eating, will very likely do more damage than good. When our daughters sense our fear or concern around food, when they sense a strong agenda with regard to what we do and don't want them to put into their mouths, their own anxiety can ramp up and their self-trust can diminish. (*What? This delicious cupcake is bad for me? Then why do I like it so much—what is wrong with me?* Or, *You're telling me I have had enough to eat? But I still feel hungry—what is wrong with me and why can't I trust my body?*)

With the best of intentions, many of us mistakenly focus on fixing immediate, short-term problems or issues such as a weight change, a disinterest in vegetables, or a love of sugar, at the expense of creating larger, long-term eating issues, including chronic dieting, inflexible palates, and food fixations. The truth is, when we try to improve one aspect of our child's health or eating (such as balancing blood sugar, reversing insulin resistance or tightly controlling the amount they a specific nutrient such as calcium, fat, protein, or sugar in their diet) without taking her overall eating well-being into account, we inadvertently damage her overall relationship with food.

By exerting overt control over small and specific aspects of our daughter's eating, such as making a certain food off-limits, forcing her to eat something we believe is healthy (but which she does not like), or telling her she hasn't eaten enough, we diminish her confidence in selecting foods, lessen the joy she feels in eating, and cause her to distrust her natural hunger. In essence, we put a ding in essential eating skills all while thinking we are doing our best to "raise a healthy eater."

The good news: By putting in some work, we can restore those skills both for daughters and for ourselves. Instead, we can take an easier approach that requires less effort and more trust. The best way to raise a happy, healthy eater is to focus on helping your daughter build one thing—eating competence.

Eating competence is not a set of rules; it's a skill that's founded in the belief that the vast majority of children have the innate ability to grow into balanced, healthy eaters. Children are born with an inner knowing that can guide them to achieve their own uniquely appropriate (not idealized) body weight.

Eating competence is not a new concept, nor is it a wishy-washy one. It is a term coined in 2007 by renowned visionary and prolific registered dietitian and family therapist Ellyn Satter after 30 years of working in the field of pediatric nutrition. According to the Ellyn Satter Institute, "eating competence is about being positive, comfortable, and flexible with eating as well as matter-of-fact and reliable about getting enough to eat of enjoyable and nourishing food."[1] In fact, since 2007, eating competence has grown into an evidenced-based and validated model of eating now referred to in clinical practice and research as ecSatter.[2] Eating competence has measurable benefits on physical, emotional, and social health.[3] Research conducted by the Satter and others shows that children (and adults!) who score high on validated measures of eating competence:

- Eat better diets that include more fruits and vegetables and higher nutritional quality

- Are more joyful and positive about eating

- Are more trusting and capable with themselves and other people

- Have the same or lower BMI

- Have better physical self-acceptance

- Are more active

- Sleep better and longer

- Have better medical profiles and lab tests

- Do better with feeding their children

In other words, eating competence is an approach towards eating that can enhance multiple aspects of a girl's well-being. It improves physical, emotional, and social health. In essence, eating competence is the key to achieving what I sense is every mother's goal—for her child to be well.

Competent eaters feel comfortable and relaxed around eating and food, they allow themselves to eat foods they enjoy, and they are flexible about foods (if a preferred food isn't available or is something they consider high fat or high sugar, they are okay eating it until a preferred food is available, for example). Competent eaters eat as much or as little as they want depending on their unique and individualized needs. They prioritize eating, making time to have meals and snacks and paying attention to their food and body during eating. (It is important to note that while eating competence is possible for many people to achieve, certain aspects of it can be more challenging than others for specific populations as you will learn later in this book. The goal is to move towards eating competence from where we are, not perfect it. It is to strive for a way of approaching eating that is more beneficial and less harmful than one that promotes eating for weight loss or dietary "perfection.")

At the core of the framework that encompasses the Intentional Feeding Mindset is the goal of developing and reinforcing eating competence. In order to create eating competence in our daughters, we need to be competent eaters ourselves. If we have a history of dieting or are at all impacted or influenced by diet culture, we can get tripped up on some of the fundamental parts of building eating competence.

For example, one major component of eating competence is permission. As described by Satter in her book *The Secrets of Feeding a Healthy Family*, eating competence is a matter of giving yourself "permission to choose food you enjoy and eat it in amounts you find satisfying." When I suggest that a mom include potato or corn chips as a side during dinner because her daughter tends to enjoy them, the conditioning that comes along with a history of dieting can make that very difficult for a her to do. Chips are considered a high-fat, low-nutrient food that feels unhealthy and unsafe—and, thus, giving herself or her daughter permission to eat them can cause some serious discomfort. What mom may not realize is that limiting chips by stowing them on a top shelf in the kitchen cabinet and regulating them to a "we really shouldn't be eating these" food can create a conflict for the child. Suddenly, the act of eating—even wanting—chips can be filled with shame and guilt. Also, a feeling of scarcity can cause kids and adults alike to go overboard when presented with the opportunity. Lastly, a handful of baked potato chips isn't that different nutritionally speaking from a scoop of mashed potatoes, making all the discomfort, conflict, and shame for naught.

In creating the concept of eating competence, Satter has divided eating skills into **four** main areas, including:

- Contextual skills, which refer to our ability to provide, plan, and prepare meals and snacks

- Eating attitudes, which include our thoughts, beliefs, and feelings about different foods

- Food acceptance, or how easily we are able to accept new foods and be flexible about foods

- Internal regulation, which is our ability to be in touch with hunger and fullness, appetite and satiety, and eat in a way that helps us maintain our body weight

The beauty of this model is that the four realms are interconnected and interdependent, which means that when we increase our daughter's skills in one area, it can *automatically* help to improve her eating skills in another area.[4] Some skills, such as internal regulation, are present from the moment we are born and we simply need to support our children in a way that allows them to stay connected (or helps them to reconnect) to those innate insights. They are what you will learn as part of our eating knowledge. Other skills, such as contextual skills, are learned and developed over time with experience and maturation. As parents, we do our best to understand the differences between these skills, as well as where we need to learn to take responsibility for our own emotions and lean out or avoid the temptation to interfere so we can allow our children to do their own work. Throughout this book, you will learn more about the four different elements of eating competence and how we can improve each over time.

By understanding more about eating competence and how to build it in our daughters, we will learn, coincidentally, how to build it in ourselves. This is a valuable byproduct that will create a virtuous cycle, meaning the more you support her, the more you support your own eating competence. And the more eating competence is strengthened within yourself, the better able you will continue to be in supporting your daughter's same set of eating competence skills.[5]

In the following chapters, we will be given opportunities to identify how our own eating histories may be impacting our attitudes and approach to feeding and talking to our daughters about eating, foods, physical activity, and weight. By building our own unique Intentional Feeding Mindset (IFM), we can overcome our roadblocks to a balanced relationship with food and give our daughter a type of confidence in her own eating that'll ensure she never faces them herself.

REFLECTIONS ON YOUR GOALS
FOR YOUR DAUGHTER

- *When it comes to reading this book, what is your goal?*

- *Why?*

- *And why is that? (Repeating the "why" question multiple times will take you deeper and deeper into the root of what you want for your daughter. Try it and see where you go.)*

- *What would that look like for you? What is the change you hope to make?*

- *What benefits do you imagine your daughter could or will enjoy by avoiding dieting altogether?*

CHAPTER THREE

INFLUENCE

"What we see, we see and seeing is changing"

—Adrienne Rich, The Fact of a Doorframe

M IRABEL'S FATHER WAS FULLY IMMERSED IN THE LIFE OF THE twelve-year-old daughter that he'd brought to see me. While that's not something I never see, I will say it's at least unusual. More often, as you might guess, mothers are the ones who step into my office. In my experience, mothers are most often involved in feeding and organizing the daily lives of their children, the ones who make the appointments with the doctors, dentists, therapists, and nutritionists, so this father struck me as interesting.

Of course, as the visit went on, my understanding of the dynamic between daughter and dad grew and I became less and less interested in what he had to say and much more interested in Mirabel's experience of her father's extraordinary attention to her eating and exercise habits. Like with most initial nutrition therapy sessions, we did a deep dive into her daily habits and routine, including what and when she eats, how often she moves, where she eats, and with whom. While dad provided many of these details, I kept trying to give her room and space to talk about it herself; unfortunately, she was not forthcoming about the minutiae of her eating life at all.

Finally, to reorient us and try to make the most of our visit, I took a step back from the food and asked her why she had decided to come to see me—what she wanted help with. Again, silence. I began to understand that Mirabel didn't want to be there at all. She stared blankly at the floor, self-conscious and guarded. Her father spoke instead.

"Mirabel has gained some weight," he said. While I knew that this young girl's BMI percentile had been increasing slightly for the past four months from her pediatrician's information, I was hoping—as I always am—that a parent can restrain themselves from making an issue of it. Or at the very least, from doing so in front of their child. Of course, asking the question is a risk, but it also creates the perfect opportunity for me to glimpse the dynamic that's going on within the family. Is this something they were openly talking about? Now I knew clearly that the answer was yes and, judging by what had happened so far—that it was *his* main concern, not necessarily hers.

Before I could respond, Mirabel interjected, "Yeah, I've been eating really unhealthy."

"What does that mean to you? What are you eating that you feel is unhealthy?" I asked, hoping to get some more of her perspective on the matter. From the intake I'd just done, she was an avocado toast for breakfast, turkey sandwich for lunch, yogurt for snack eating kind of gal. With three days of two-hour-long swim practices listed, among a host of other recreational physical activity, I was wondering how she was surviving on so little to eat.

"Bubble tea. And sometimes hamburgers and French fries. I usually eat that when I go out with my friends," she said. Her father nodded somberly in agreement. He disapproved.

"Well, I'm not sure that's necessarily a problem," I started. "I'll have to do some more calculations, but from what you've shared with me so far, I was thinking you probably need some extra calories. A snack after school makes sense." I glanced at dad, unsurprised that he was uncomfortable with that information. And in the silence, I looked back at her only to notice that she was crying.

As I handed her a box of tissues, she started telling me about her belly and how she hates it. "All my friends have Instagram accounts and post photos of their flat bellies," she said between deep and unsure breaths. I acknowledged her sadness and stress, tried weakly to point out how superficial it is to value someone because of the flatness of their belly, questioned whether that was a quality she looked for in friends, then pointed out the fact that she was a beautiful girl who had a perfectly healthy body, and it was a shame that she'd ever waste her time not liking it. I was waiting during the awkward silences for her father to rush in with his own reassurance, or at least consternation about the fact that she'd been using social media to beat herself up. In my opinion, he was doing way too little to console her.

In the absence of his comfort, I acknowledged that being a teen can be really tough, then asked her if she had anyone to talk to about it. She said, "No. I'd talk to my mom, but she's always so busy with work and it's hard for her to listen and she's always mad at me," came out all in one breath. It was a knife to my own heart; a conflict I was having with my own daughter at home.

Minutes later, with Mirabel out of the room, I tried to feel out dad. Had he been encouraging her to diet? "No, her mom and I just want her to eat healthy," he explained. He was understandably defensive. When I asked him if he knew that she had these social media accounts and that she and her friends had been posting pics of their bodies, he said yes, he did. She had cried to him about it, too, which explained his indecipherable level of reaction to hearing about it moments earlier.

"She *does* have a belly," he told me, as if to explain that she *does*, in fact, need to stop gaining weight. "Listen, her mother and I know not to tell her to go on a diet. My wife is a feminist and our friends have a daughter with an eating disorder," he shared. "We just want her to take better care of herself. We want her to be healthy. And she's not happy with the way her body looks right now," he emphasized. "And she has too much after school already to start up with a therapist."

As far as I was concerned, a lecture about the importance of eating for weight control from a nutritionist was the last thing Mirabel needed. A better understanding of the complex set of influences—diet culture, family values, weight stigma and weight-centered healthcare, and body changes associated with puberty—that were deceptively causing her parents to recommend dieting to their daughter would be better.

All names and identifying details of my patients have been changed to protect client-patient confidentiality.

UNDERSTANDING INFLUENCE STRENGTHENS OUR IFM

The things that influence our approach to eating, our attitudes towards food, and our regard for our body are complex, sometimes in contradiction to one another, and can be difficult to call out or identify. In this chapter, you will learn to identify some of the forces that may be impacting how both you and your daughter think and feel about food, body, and health. Going forward, this information will help you avoid clouding your judgment or being swayed from your original goal and intentions for your daughter.

When you are faced with a tough situation or question regarding your daughter's eating (or not eating)—for example, your mother keeps expressing her "concern" about your daughter's portion sizes, your daughter insists she needs to diet because she'll be happier if she's thinner, or you're wondering if that extra layer of fat your daughter recently developed around her belly really is a problem to address—you'll have a better perspective on what might be influencing them, her, and your own thoughts. With a deeper understanding of these influences in mind, it'll be easier to know how to best intervene in a positive and effective way.

IFM Touchstone: *Influence*

As you read this chapter, try to identify which source of influence is most at play in your daughter's life when it comes to her relationship with food and her body. If it is harmful, what is one small action you can take to protect her from it? For example, *I intend to limit my social media use to x minutes per day, I intend to remind myself that gaining fat during puberty is healthy and normal,* or *I intend to talk to my sister-in-law about avoiding diet talk at the table before our next dinner together.*

INFLUENCE OF OUR OWN VALUES

On many occasions, I have had parents tell me that they don't know why their daughter is dieting or why she is so concerned about her weight. They insist that their daughter is healthy and perfect just as she is and, many times, I've had the pleasure of witnessing parents happily and genuinely reassure their children of such things. Yet, in the same conversations, parents also share things such as, "We eat really healthy," "I've always watched what I eat," and "I work out every morning." What I don't think these well-meaning parents realize is that even when we aren't overtly telling our daughters they need to lose weight, we may still be sending them the message that we place high value on certain standards of eating and physical activity. And, thanks to diet culture, the subtext that our daughters are likely picking up is that we are doing these things because we also value being a certain body shape, size, or weight.

We all need to be aware of how we ourselves are influenced by diet and health culture, as well as how we might pass those influences on to our daughters. Sometimes, it requires us to look more deeply into ourselves and our habits, including our own relationship to food, body, weight, and activity.

For example, are we promoting eating more fruits and vegetables to our kids because we know these foods support our immune system or because we know that are low in calories? (Perhaps a little of both, I suspect.) Are we explaining that being active is important to us because it helps us manage stress, or are we allowing our kids to assume that we are "staying in shape" to help us manipulate our weight? Since there is so much opportunity for our daughters to internalize that latter motivation, I think it is important to clarify our intentions at every opportunity to avoid inadvertently passing along misaligned values. Here are some strategies for clarifying our own values to our daughters, which will help you create a stronger, more effective, and explicit IFM.

Ask Her about Healthy Eating. Give your daughter an opportunity to tell you what she thinks "healthy eating" means. Then check in on it again as often as you see fit, as her ideas may change as she's exposed to new influences. You might be surprised at what you hear. If your daughter, like many of the pre-teens and teens I have worked with, equates "healthy eating" with restrictive eating styles such as veganism or only eating low-carb foods, then when we tell them we want them to be "healthy eaters," we may be greenlighting a diet without even realizing it. In addition, when girls tell me they want to be "healthy" and I've asked what that means, I've gotten answers like "not being obese" and "it means you work out all the time." These same girls also express shame for not living up to these incorrect ideals. When you ask your daughter what she thinks "healthy eating" means, you get an opportunity to correct any inaccuracies or misinformation. If your daughter's answer was off or unsettling, then you know to take extra care to be clear about what you value with regard to eating habits (eating food prepared at home, eating together, eating intuitively, for example, as opposed to the healthy diet *du jour*, such as keto) when you talk with her about food in the future.

Step Off the Scale. If we are stepping on a scale regularly, then we are sending her a subtle yet powerful message that, to us, body weight is important—even without mentioning the word weight at all. If weight weren't important to us, why else would you be measuring it? For most parents, I recommend removing the scale from the home entirely. From conversations I've had with adolescent and teenage clients, even if you feel you're being discrete about weighing yourself, there's a good chance your daughter knows you're doing it. There's also a good chance your daughter is using it to measure her own weight, even if you keep the scale tucked away in your closet or bathroom and openly discourage it. More than once, a parent has answered "never" when I ask during an intake how often their daughter has been weighing herself, only to find out the answer is closer to "weekly" or even "daily" when I talk to the girl herself.

Many parents have also expressed feeling uncomfortable with getting rid of their scale, particularly if weighing themselves is a habit they've had for years. (If that's you, I encourage you to ask yourself a few questions: *What is the purpose of measuring my weight? What do I do if the number is higher than expected? What if it is lower? How is the information helping me? How might it be harming me?* In my experience, that number can set off a cascade of emotions that can negatively impact self-esteem and eating and exercise behaviors in some people. Not everyone, but some. I encourage you to check in with where you're at with feelings about your weight.) For parents who do decide to keep the scale in the home, I also always recommend they avoid weighing themselves in front of their children. And if you have a medical reason to be weighing yourself daily (if you're taking a medication that's dosed by weight or have kidney or heart disease, for example), make it known that you don't believe weight is a measure of health or personal virtue. In other words, I think it's worth being extra clear about where you stand on this particular topic to counter any message you may otherwise be sending.

Be Clear on Activity. If you invest a lot of time in exercise, physical activity, or being at the gym, be clear on why you're doing it. Take it as an opportunity to promote the multiple benefits of *movement* (explained in Chapter 9) over any intention to keep or correct your figure, repent for food eaten, or even because it's important to be fit (which again could be construed as meaning being thin, if you don't clarify that for her). When mothers talk about their own eating and activity efforts as ways to be healthy or increase their fitness, as opposed to weight loss, their daughters are less likely to diet and are happier with their own bodies.[1]

Unlink Eating and Weight. When you do talk about healthy eating, avoid referencing weight altogether.[2] In families where parents talk about "weight" (including eating to maintain weight or avoid gaining weight), kids have more disordered eating habits (such as restrictive eating and binge eating), lower self-esteem, more body dissatisfaction, and are more likely to be depressed. This is regardless of whether they are raising a child who is considered underweight, normal weight, or overweight.[3] Those negative effects are powerful and have been shown to last at least 15 years, following kids into adulthood.[4] What's better? Focusing conversations on what researchers called "healthful" eating—eating meals that include a mix of nutrients, or talking about the benefits of foods on our energy, growth, or blood sugar. When parents make this slight reframe to their food talk, it makes a positive and powerful difference, including lowering the risk of disordered eating and increasing fruit and vegetable intake. If you get tongue-tied or the stakes feel just too high at meal times and you still "worry I'm going to say the wrong thing," as multiple moms have told me, try this: just don't say anything. Focus on enjoying your child's company and initiate pleasant topics of conversation instead.

Ditching Your Own Diet. As you probably suspect, when parents focus on their own weight loss attempts, their children are more likely to be dissatisfied with their bodies and weight as well, and may try dieting themselves.[5] The effect is particularly strong for those parents who used more extreme, noticeable, and restrictive weight-loss strategies, such as skipping meals, compared to those who used less obvious ones, such as eating a smaller portion at dinner. Not surprisingly, the converse has also been shown to be true. When parents—mothers in particular—rarely or never talk of their own weight struggles, their daughter's own desire to be thinner and to diet was significantly lower, too.[6]

If you have been on a diet or fretted about your weight in front of your daughter in the past, stop worrying or feeling guilty about it. First, you know better now. Second, no *one* thing we as mothers have done or not done is ever responsible for how our daughters behave around food or feel about their body (or anything else, for that matter). And third, the fact that you're reading this book is an excellent indicator that you're working hard to create as positive an environment as possible for your daughter in terms of food and body. Frankly, I'm not sure of what better thing you could do to counter any concerns you may have about her relationship with food! If you find yourself talking about your own eating or exercising routines, again, be sure to frame it as a way to meet your goal of staying healthy in specific, non-weight-related ways (for example, to balance blood sugar, increase energy) or improving your fitness level to reach an enjoyable goal (say by getting stronger or increasing your endurance in order to complete a challenging hike, join a walk or run for charity or improve your tennis game).

INFLUENCE OF FAMILY

Even when we set the course for positive body image and a healthy relationship with food for our daughters, inevitably another well-meaning family member comes along and rocks the boat. Diet and health culture are so pervasive, that any one of us would be hard-pressed to say that there's no live wire in our family that we need to worry about when it comes to a conversation with their own dieting or weight-based rhetoric. In fact, sometimes they aim the comments directly at our daughters, or the comments come from someone who made similar comments towards us as a child. (Honestly, I've been in both situations, and I can't say which stings worse!)

Never fear. Whether it's a blood relative, in-law, a person you've known forever, or even your own children, there are ways to protect your daughter from in-the-house influencers who comment on her weight, what she has on her plate, how much or how little she eats, or how her body has changed since they last saw her. Here are four things to keep in mind before you fire back at a family member who threatens to make your daughter feel bad about her eating.

1. ***Know Your Goal.*** Before you respond, remind yourself of the reason that you're saying something in the first place. This will up the odds that you'll get the outcome you want. For example, my goals are to help my daughters have a happy, healthy relationship with food and body, to ensure they enjoy eating, feel at ease at meals, and stay in touch with their innate ability to self-regulate. It is *not* to erase decades of "thinner is better" programming from the minds of my relatives, nor is it to educate anyone on the problem with weight-centric healthcare, nor to outline the impact of patriarchy on women's feelings about their appetites and their bodies. Those things are all important to me, I just choose not to work on them at the dinner table because I feel it distracts from the safe, peaceful eating environment I want for my daughters.

2. ***Know Your Audience.*** Before you respond to comments that make you uncomfortable, take a second to think about who you're speaking to. This is a tip I learned from Virgie Tovar, an author, fat-activist, and host of the podcast Rebel Eaters Club. Based on what you already know about this person, ask yourself, *Does this person tend to be rigid in their thoughts and thinking? Do they seem to shut you down and ignore your opinion and perspective? Or are they more flexible, open-minded, and responsive to information I share?* If the family member or friend in question is difficult and rigid, I recommend making a clear and

firm boundary as soon as you feel your daughter's eating-esteem is at stake. If mom or mother-in-law (MIL) says, "I think you've had enough" to your daughter, you can say for example, "We have a rule about not commenting on how much or how little each other eats." If she says, "It looks like you're gaining weight," you can say "We don't comment on other people's bodies." If it continues to happen, privately explain that if she breaks the rule or disagrees with it, then you will not be able to eat meals together. Harsh? Yes. Necessary? In my opinion, very much yes!

If you're blessed enough to have family members who are more open, curious, and sensitive to your thoughts and perspective, you might share some of your reasons for the rules or boundaries you set. "We have this rule because I have had a difficult time dieting my whole life and I want to make sure that my daughter doesn't." Or, "We don't comment on the food because we know it will have a negative impact on her eating." Explaining personal reasons can make the rule more meaningful and compelling, which will increase the chances someone will agree with and respect it.

The rules you set can go for comments that cross lines with body types and even negative feelings about their own eating, too. For example, if your uncle continually shares that his new keto diet is helping him slim down and "get skinny," you can politely tell him that you don't talk about dieting in front of your children. If your sister is lamenting about how "disgusting" she feels because she ate too much cake, you can tell her talking negatively about her body makes your girls feel guilty about eating cake, too, so please stop. If your college-age niece shares that she feels "fat," you can say, "My girls know 'fat' is a beautiful thing that protects our bodies and that women typically have more of it than men! They know you have 'fat' on your body, and they know you are smart, funny, and strong." Whatever you opt for, fill in your own values and boundaries—just be direct, clear, and positive to get the best results.

3. ***Take Immediate Positive Action.*** As a pre-teen obsessing about my weight, I couldn't imagine anything more positive and powerful than the image of my older cousin slicing herself a giant piece of our family's favorite cheesecake immediately following a dinner table discussion about how many grams of sugar were in several different types of desserts. She sent a silent signal to everyone at the table that she couldn't care less about a word of what they said—and to a girl who admired her and had been taught nothing but the virtue of food restraint, it was downright beautiful.

While many of the comments and confrontations you might have will need to be done in private and away from your young daughter, taking positive action in the moment is also important. Sometimes it might be to deflect, minimize, or pivot the conversation, and sometimes it will be to confront and neutralize the negativity. Simply changing the subject can be positive and proactive, too, in my opinion.

Recently, for instance, friends we see just once or twice a year started talking to my husband about how much body fat their adolescent daughter had packed on during COVID compared to other girls in her class. Before I passed out in horror, I sliced through their conversation with, "Are we going to get outside with the kids now or what?" Poof! It was over. Other times, I've taken more direct action, either by putting up a boundary (or restating it if it's been an ongoing issue) or responding with something deliberately contrary and positive such as in all the examples above. Just because I'm not up for starting a heavy debate about diet culture or weight, doesn't mean I recommend staying or being silent. Letting uncomfortable things lie with people you're close with doesn't help your daughter. If we want to teach her to advocate for herself with regard to these issues—such as having full say over what and how much she eats—then the most powerful way to help her is by being brave enough to do it ourselves. If this isn't your natural style, start in a safe place—say, with a close friend or relative with whom you have a more playful or light relationship with. For example, the last time my brother said, "Are you really going to have another slice of cake?" I used it as an opportunity to make sure both my daughters heard me respond, "Absolutely. And don't ever comment on what I eat again." I flashed both of my girls a big smile so that so they understood that it's possible to assert yourself without being hostile, and maybe even having some fun.

4. ***Consider How Frequently You Eat Together.*** Confronting a parenting partner or another caregiver who eats many or all meals with your daughter will require a different tactic than a person who is related but has less say or sway over your child's eating. For co-parents and anyone else who feeds your daughter or with whom she eats regularly, I'd recommend a longer, more intimate discussion of your concerns. (For tips on talking to a co-parent, visit the NourishHer.com/blog.)

INFLUENCE OF DIET CULTURE

When I went back to school to study nutrition as a second career in 2011, diet culture was not a topic we read or talked about. That seems odd, in retrospect, given the fact that diet culture shapes so many of our beliefs about food and health and, therefore, our eating. Today, diet culture is being called out, discussed, and criticized by an ever-increasing number of dietitians and healthcare professionals. That's great news, since recognizing diet culture is one of the key steps to reducing its incessant influence on us and our daughters. This entire book, in fact, exists as a tool to help combat diet culture, and many of the influences called out in this chapter are deeply rooted in diet culture. (And I know that you, my warrior mother, are likely already well aware of its impact.) However, in this section we'll get a chance to deepen our understanding of what diet culture really is—and learn about the sneaky ways it comes right up onto our dinner table—to help lessen its influence even further.

While there's no official definition of the term "diet culture," anti-diet activist and dietitian Harrison (who I mentioned earlier nicknamed it the "Life Thief") does a lovely job describing it. According to her, diet culture is "a system of beliefs that equates thinness, muscularity, and particular body shapes with health and moral virtue; promotes weight loss and body reshaping as a means of attaining higher status; demonizes certain foods and food groups while elevating others; and oppresses people who don't match its supposed picture of 'health.'

"By and large, Western culture is diet culture. This way of thinking about food and bodies is so embedded in the fabric of our society, in so many different forms, that it can be hard to recognize," says Harrison. Her definition of diet culture will definitely resonate with those of us who have felt or are feeling burdened (or, in some moments, downright destroyed) by the pressure to be thin.

Diet culture is that perpetual pressure to be thin that seems to underlie everything. It's what is at the root of jaw-dropping phenomena and statistics, such as five-year-old girls being worried about their weight, 45 percent of 16-to-19-year-old girls being on a diet, and young girls' fear of the potential of being fat as a significant driver in the development of an eating disorder.[7]

Diet culture can be large, loud, and in our face—for example, a billboard advertising for a new weight loss supplement. It can also be a subtle suggestion we've been following for years, such as drinking a glass of water ahead of time to make sure you don't eat so much at a meal. And when we can't walk the aisle of our favorite market without seeing a new food with the word "skinny" in it, well that's diet culture, too.

Diet culture is perpetuated by the medical system, which determines health status (and so often consciously or unconsciously, moral virtue) to people based on BMI. (For more information on how to unravel the connection between weight and health, see Chapter 5.) And from my perspective, to be a dietitian aware of the dangers of diet culture and someone who works within a major medical system is to walk a very, very fine line indeed!

Diet culture exists because of anti-fat bias. Whether we are willing to admit it or not, Diet culture can then be considered a social justice issue because the anti-fat bias that under pins it does more than just wreak havoc at our dinner table. It contributes to bias and stigma and causes negative impacts on overall well-being, including multiple elements of physical, emotional, and social health. Diet culture (or its anti-fat root) contributes to health disparities and disproportionately impacts women, people in larger bodies, people of non-dominant cultures, ethnicities, or races, people of the LGBTQ+ community, and people of lower socioeconomic status who are experiencing food insecurity. Diet culture can be at times one or all of the following: elitist, classist, misogynistic, and racist. It's heavy stuff with big implications that go beyond our individual relationships with food or how we eat.

Here's the sneaky way that diet culture hoodwinks us, interfering with our relationship with food even when we're *not* trying to lose weight. Diet culture tightly intertwines our notion of good health with thinness, so without even realizing it we equate raising our kids to be healthy eaters to mean we also raise them to eat in a way that keeps (or makes) their bodies meet cultural ideals of thinness. Diet culture crosses the giant chasm between eating to be thin and eating to be healthy, making us believe that they are one and the same.

Diet culture has in so many ways become health culture that's it tough to escape. As Harrison believes, you'd be hard-pressed to find a person living in the U.S. who hasn't been impacted by the ideas and attitudes that come from the constant pressure to be "healthy." In other words, I consider the pressure we feel to be and raise "healthy" eaters as an insidious and not-so-obvious form of diet culture. In effect, we believe that "healthy" eaters are thin people.

Diet culture's intersection with healthism and what I call "food parenting culture" is what creates all kinds of undue stress, frustration, self-judgment, and worry for us as parents even when we are adamant that we don't condone dieting or weight loss for our kids.

It's the blurred line between dieting and healthy eating that can make eating with our kids feel stressful, confusing, and at times even heart-wrenching. The unclear difference between eating to avoid weight gain and eating to be healthy presents problems meal after meal, snack after snack, and special occasion after special occasion. Disguised as a concern for health, weight-centric concerns are so ingrained in our approach to eating they push us to question whether it's okay to give in to the simplest of our daughter's food needs. For example, we get uneasy when they ask for second or third helpings of noodles or bread wondering if we should dissuade them or simply say no. Or we feel tense and frustrated by their natural love of sweet foods like candy, cake, cookies, or dessert. We also feel disappointed and overly concerned when they don't take the same interest in uber "healthy" (i.e., low calorie) foods like vegetables. Latent fears about weight gain—veiled as worry about whether a choice is healthy—make us feel guilty for letting our child order the pasta (again), judged for picking up a fast-food meal in a time pinch, or apologetic for putting a premade, packaged food in her lunchbox.

When diet culture co-opts the meaning of healthy eating, it also has the power to make us and our daughters believe those who make food choices such as organic, locally grown, natural, non-GMO; or eating styles such as "clean," low-carb, keto, paleo, vegan and vegetarianism are smarter, healthier, and destined-to-be-thin people because of it—and guilty or bad when we can't keep up or follow suit.

All these terribly complicated things aside, there is some good news for parents. Focusing on developing **eating competence** can undermine the negative influence of diet culture on your and your children's relationship with food.

For example, checking in with your attitudes towards foods such as which foods are good for you and which aren't (which we will do in the chapter on nutrition) can help erase some of the healthy vs unhealthy food myths that diet culture helped to create. Focusing on the structure and timing of meals is more effective at helping kids eat and enjoy balanced, healthy foods as opposed to wiping your house clean of what diet culture considers totally "off-limits" food. Building internal regulation skills with approaches such as intuitive eating can help you and your child maintain a more stable (i.e., healthier) body weight as opposed to using painful diet culture tactics to outsmart your hunger. And learning to prepare foods in delicious, satisfying ways can help you and your daughter learn to like new foods as opposed to opting for the low-calorie preparation styles (and expensive gadgets) diet culture pressures us to use.

In other words, the eating and feeding skills you're learning in this book can help your daughter build a solid foundation and good defense against the unrelenting influence of diet culture and a health-at-all-costs mentality creates.

> **Bookmark** *Anti-Diet: Reclaim Your Time, Money, Well-Being, and Happiness Through Intuitive Eating* by Christy Harrison, MPH, RD. In her book, you can learn about the history of dieting, get insights into using intuitive eating as a solution for creating healthier relationships with food, and deepen your perspective on diet culture from a social justice perspective.

INFLUENCE OF WEIGHT STIGMA

A few years ago, I sat around a conference table with a group of pediatric endocrinologists that I had been working with for a few years and presented a short nutrition lecture called "How to Talk to Parents About Weight." The surprising reaction to my presentation changed the course of my career.

Knowing the best ways to discuss the delicate issue of weight with families is a task most pediatric endocrinologists are faced with daily. What I had intended to share were the most effective and supportive ways to talk to parents and children about the daily habits they might incorporate into their routine to help with whatever particular dysfunction they were being seen for (such as diabetes or insulin resistance), as opposed to focusing on their body weight. Some of the habits I wanted to share, for example, included eating fiber-containing foods, avoiding sugary beverages, getting sufficient daily activity and sleep, and having family meals together. I also wanted to share how their choice of words could help their patients, too, as recent findings at that time showed that parents raising children in larger bodies prefer when their providers use the term "BMI" to "overweight" or "obese" when talking about their child's weight. What I was not there to do was convince them to avoid talking about weight with kids altogether. Naively, I assumed they were already doing their best to avoid focusing on a child's body weight when talking to families, given the risks of encouraging weight loss and dieting, particularly in the case of children. Those risks, including triggering disordered eating and eating disorders, tend to be interpreted as a recommendation to diet, which has (ironically) been shown to increase overall body weight in children and increase the harmful effects of weight stigma that children in larger bodies (and often their parents) are often already experiencing.

Unfortunately, that talk was more of a learning experience for *me* than for them.

As it turned out, the crowd could not move past the underlying assumption of my talk, which was that weight itself might not be the problem everyone has long understood it to be, nor should we be discussing it directly with families and children. By the time I was done talking, just one third-year fellow expressed interest in knowing more about how to talk to parents and children in non-stigmatizing ways. The rest of the providers wanted to double back and talk about *why* they should avoid talking about weight and avoiding weight gain in the first place.

For the majority of people, weight stigma still needs a lecture of its own. Despite prestigious organizations such as the American Academy of Pediatrics and medical journals such as *The Lancet* publishing policy papers and research initiatives on the significant harms of weight bias and stigma, I continue to be surprised about how many people in healthcare are still hesitant to acknowledge how utterly detrimental emphasizing weight as a problem—and weight loss as a solution—can be to people's health and well-being.

If I could rewind time and erase that presentation I gave to my colleagues, I would start fresh with a new one about how our own bias against larger bodies impacts our ability to provide compassionate and effective healthcare. I would have done better to take a few steps back and present research that countered the strongly held belief that larger bodies and higher BMIs are problems in and of themselves that need to be fixed. That strongly held paradigm—despite years of evidence proving it wrong and despite the fact that it causes significant harm to millions of people—is one that a large part of the medical community remains unable to shift.[e] I would have talked about the ways in which the weight stigma and fat phobia that runs rampant in traditional healthcare harms everyone, regardless of their BMI or weight.

So what is weight stigma and how does it influence our daughters and the people who care for them? Weight stigma is the bias we feel or discrimination we show towards people living in larger bodies. People who feel stigmatized due to their body weight suffer from social, emotional, and even physical consequences. Stigmatized individuals are more likely to be socially isolated, less likely to be active, more likely to binge eat, less likely to seek out medical care, and less likely to partake in physical activity, which can further contribute to poor health outcomes, and increased feelings of isolation.[9] Adolescents who internalize weight bias are more likely to have lower self-esteem and engage in binge and emotional eating.[10] Weight stigma decreases people's quality of life, particularly in children.[11] Weight stigma is powerful and kids pick up early on the idea that being in a bigger body might be a problem; researchers have detected it in children as young as three.[12] With these risks in mind, when healthcare providers focus on our daughters' weight and perpetuate weight stigma, they are not helping; they are harming. They're worsening the very outcomes they are hoping to improve.

The stigmatizing effects of being in a body that's large, has a certain higher BMI set point, or has visible or excessive fat stores causes a fear of fatness for everyone. Some research shows that it's a fear of fatness, not necessarily a drive for thinness, that drives young girls' desire to diet, for example.[13]

Another way weight stigma causes harm? When providers are blinded by BMI, meaning they see a larger body as a problem and then attribute whatever health complaints an adult or child may have to weight, without taking the opportunity to dig deeper, find, and treat the real cause of a health condition. For example, a provider might a symptom that a fatter-than-average child complains of such as worsening asthma on the patient's weight, as opposed to asking about other possible causes for the change in their condition, such as being newly exposed to mold or chemicals. Or they may assume that an adolescent who has gained a significant amount of weight is eating too many chips or candy and offer "healthy eating" advice as opposed to screening them for an eating disorder or food insecurity.

Unfortunately, shame is the name of the game when it comes to weight stigma. The American Academy of Pediatrics points out that, despite knowing that it causes harm, one reason weight stigma continues in the medical field is because many people believe that shaming people in larger bodies is a good way to motivate them to lose weight.[11] (Yes, this is true. And I can hardly believe it myself.)

Unfortunately, the influence of weight stigma and fat phobia on kids and adults extends well beyond healthcare (and is beyond the scope of this book). However, for the purpose of protecting your daughter from dieting, and since I think you have a good chance of advocating for her in this particular arena, I do want to zero in on the doctor's office. I believe we need to be particularly aware of the influence of weight stigma when we seek medical care (regardless of our daughter's weight) if we want them to have happy, healthy relationships with food and their body, for the following reasons:

Weight-Centered Care is Everywhere. First, since our current medical system is rooted in weight-based care, it means that most physicians are trained to see weight as a core feature of your child's health. A doctor's office is a place where your child's well-being will be judged (or *assessed*, to use a clinical term) based on body measurements, particularly their BMI percentile. We want to avoid that perspective from influencing how our girls feel about themselves, their bodies, eating, or overall health.

UNDERSTANDING BMI PERCENTILE.

This number compares a child's BMI to other children of the same age and gender. So, for example, a BMI of 65 means a child has a BMI that is greater than 65 percent of girls the same age. When looking at a child's BMI, it is important to track changes over time, as opposed to getting caught up on where that number falls in comparison to other children. For example, a BMI percentile of 90 can be perfectly normal and healthy, particularly if that is the same percentile the child has been tracking for years, while a BMI percentile of 50 could be a problem if your daughter had been consistently tracking much higher, for example.

MD Signals Authority. Second, doctors have incredible sway and influence over their patients. In the case of impressionable children who may already feel self-conscious and vulnerable because of their weight, a doctor's influence may even be greater. In listening to stories from my adult patients and reading multiple heated and emotion-laden threads on social media and blog articles from women well into their 20s, 30s, and 40s, a negative word about weight from a medical doctor has been known to have devasting and long-lasting impacts, including being cited as a trigger for an eventual eating disorder. If your child's pediatrician has a concern or opinion about your child's eating habits, weight, or disease risk, it's best they share that with you in private. Then you can share with your daughter what you feel is relevant, non-damaging, and appropriate.

Our Stress Strengthens Their Influence. Third, not only do doctors themselves have certain authority that has a powerful influence over us and our children, there's also evidence that the circumstances under which we are given those recommendations can make them even more pronounced in our minds. When we are under heightened stress, for example, as we might be during a medical visit, any information we hear tends to get imprinted on the brain in a significant way. That means, if you're in a scary or stressful medical situation with a valid concern and a provider then comments on your daughter's weight or makes recommendations about what she should or shouldn't be eating, you and she, if she's within earshot, are going to take that advice as gospel.

I've witnessed this firsthand while working in the hospital. When I was working with the parents of a child who'd just been diagnosed with Type 1 diabetes, I found that anything that was said to them about how to care for their child during the first day or two of diagnosis was nearly impossible to erase—including misinformation. If a nurse told them that the best way to balance their child's blood sugar was to remove carbohydrates from their diet completely, it took an incredible amount of re-education and multiple reassurances to convince them of anything different.

Kids Hear Recommendations Differently. If your daughter gets a recommendation from her pediatrician to "watch her weight" or "start eating a little healthier," it may be interpreted differently from how it was meant. "Kids don't have an ability to take a nuanced approach to weight loss; they are more black-and-white thinkers, so if a doctor tells them their BMI is high and then a family member reinforces that message that their weight or eating is a problem, they tend to make giant sweeping changes. They tend to pursue weight loss at any cost, such as cutting calories dramatically or cutting out entire food groups," explains Tracy Richmond, MD, MPH, director of the Eating Disorder Program at Boston Children's Hospital. "Young children in particular don't yet have the ability to take the long-term view regarding weight loss and will pursue extreme changes all at once."

MDs Are Pressed for Time. As a registered dietitian providing nutrition counseling, I have the luxury of taking an extensive amount of research into a family's habits before I offer any education or information around eating or activity. That means I offer recommendations *in the context of everything else* that is already going on with that child's eating and growth. A doctor assessing weight in the context of a medical visit does not have that same luxury of knowing all their eating habits and food attitudes or their history with disordered eating or dieting, thus their well-meaning recommendations to "eat more vegetables" or "move more" might be off and even harmful. If, for example, your daughter is already eating a balanced diet and is active, it will at the very least confuse her or undermine her already healthy habits, since it's been inadvertently implied that they are not enough. I once had a tenth grader and her mother come to me for weight management at the advice of both her endocrinologist and liver specialists. During the initial assessment, I discovered she'd been exercising nearly four hours per day—three hours in the evenings for her crew team and then running laps around a track during a free period at school. After hearing from two doctors that her elevated BMI was putting her at risk for diabetes and liver disease, convincing her that she needed to almost triple the number of calories compared to what she'd dropped it down to in order to meet energy needs, it felt nearly impossible. It's not unusual for a person to fall into the medical community considers an "obese" BMI percentile while also being extremely fit and active. In this young woman's case, the reasons were two-fold.

First, while I never did have a chance to assess her body fat percentage during our virtual visits, I had an inkling it was low due to her and her mother's comments about the "muscularity" of her body—and her legs, in particular. Muscle weighs more than fat, and athletes often have BMIs that range far above what the mainstream medical community labels "healthy." (Not surprisingly, while I was happy to share with this fact with her, it was difficult to convince the teen of its truth.) Additionally, her BMI, like most children's, was being assessed against the Centers for Disease Control measures and therefore wasn't taking into account her race nor the physical characteristics and body type that go with it.

Additionally, if a provider praises your daughter's drop in BMI percentile (from an "overweight" category to a "healthy weight" category) without taking stock of the dietary or activity changes she used to accomplish the drop, they might inadvertently promote or reinforce any harmful and disordered habits she used, such as skipping meals, cutting out food groups, or overexercising.

Our Perceptions Can Be Off. You may be wondering why I say we all have to be on guard for weight stigma at the doctor's office regardless of our daughters' body weights. Research shows that parents are notoriously poor judges of their daughter's weight, in some cases seeing them as being much heavier (and thus, unhealthier) than they are, as was the case with Mirabel, while others see them as thinner than they are.[13] While the latter may be protecting you from stigma in one sense, it can also leave you vulnerable. I've seen many parents blindsided at a medical visit when a provider, who is armed with a very precise measuring device, shares their child's height, weight, and BMI percentile as well as their opinion of it.

SKINNY GIRLS' BODIES GET CRITICIZED TOO.

While our culture is more fat-phobic than thin-adverse, if your daughter or another one of your children are regarded as a skinny kid, you may have noticed that people tend to make comments about their body and assumptions about their eating habits too. Having worked for years with children at both sides of the BMI spectrum, I can share with you that those at lower than "healthy weight" BMI categories often feel judged, self-conscious, and insecure about their bodies when they are being evaluated at their medical visits. If your child is particularly thin, that criticism can have similarly negative impacts on their body esteem and their eating. With that in mind, I think we can be proactive about protecting our kids from weight talk, regardless of what side of the spectrum they fall.

The bottom line is this: whatever edicts and recommendations—off-the-cuff or otherwise—that are given during a medical visit or while in a high stress, health-related situation (which I pray you never experience) carry significantly more weight than what's read in a book or shared by a friend.

While I don't recommend ignoring or being closed off to the information or weigh-ins completely—in fact, they are still necessary—I do recommend you consider offering some protection for your daughter from stigmatizing language and views on health. If you agree and choose to do so, here are some tips that may be helpful.

POSITIVE WAYS TO HANDLE WEIGH-INS AT THE PEDIATRICIAN

- *Don't Refuse Them Altogether.* You can decline weigh-ins for sick day visits and other non-annual visits. However, it is important to get at least an annual measure of your daughter's height and weight so the pediatrician can evaluate her growth. Those measurements may need to be taken even more frequently if she is being seen for a growth-related condition, taking a medication that is dosed by weight, or undergoing weight restoration for an eating disorder, for example. A significant drop in weight or decrease in BMI percentile could alert you to a problem, such as a growth disturbance or pattern of disordered eating (i.e., extreme or long-term food restriction) that you might otherwise be unaware of.

- *Ask for Blind Weigh-ins.* If and when your daughter does need to be measured, you can ask that a "blind weight" be taken, which means that your child will be facing away from the number on the scale and it will only be documented in the chart as opposed to shared openly with her.

- *Call Ahead.* Ahead of a doctor visit, ask that a note be put in your child's chart that says, "I do not consent to my child's weight, height, or growth being discussed with her. If you have concerns about any of these measurements, please discuss them with me privately." Since a note in the chart might get overlooked by a medical assistant and a nurse will likely do the measuring, you can reiterate this privately to them ahead of walking into an exam room. Once you hear any of the providers in private, you can choose how and if to share them with your daughter at your own discretion. Depending on the age of your child, you may also be able to take positive, health-protecting action—by offering more opportunity for movement or switching up the content or frequency with which you offer snacks and meals, at your own discretion.

INFLUENCE OF MEDIA

Just a few months into working as a pediatric dietitian, I noticed an interesting similarity in the way many parents would start our initial consultation. Before we'd even get into the details of what their child was eating, they would start off by making what felt like an apology or shameful confession. With their heads down, they'd say, "Well, we don't always eat organic" or, "I don't always make things from scratch" or, "I'm sorry, but I really don't like kale." The truth, though I didn't yet have the confidence to share it, was that neither did I.

Parents are almost always aware of the fact that advertising, books, movies, and social media sway us when it comes to pursuing the thin ideal. What they may not realize is how much media also influences the way we feel about other aspects of our lives as mothers, such as our cooking, food parenting skills, and our daughters' eating habits. In some cases, following the advice of a fellow mommy influencer in the media can help us feel better about ourselves in these areas—and sometimes it can ratchet up self-criticism and fear.[14]

Is one blogger being helpful when she shares that she started avoiding foods grown with fertilizers and pesticides because she thinks its healthier? Not if it means you start cutting back on fruits and vegetables because you're now skeptical of regular produce and organic is too expensive. Can making foods from scratch be better than picking up take-out? Not if there are days when you don't have the time, energy, or money that it takes to cook. Is kale a leafy green that's loaded with beneficial vitamins and antioxidants? Yes; but not liking or wanting to cook it for your kids isn't something to feel bad about.

If you find yourself following influencers on social, reading blogs, or investing in best-selling books that feature beautifully balanced meals and snacks prepared in the peaceful environment of a clean, wide open, white kitchen, then you are exposing yourself to a strong source of influence on you and on your family's food preferences and eating. Despite what feel like helpful, inspiring ideas for breakfasts, lunches, and dinners that promise to elevate your family's health and happiness to a whole a new level, the truth remains: You don't *need* to cook with only high-end, organic, GMO-free, fair trade, exotic, and (mostly) expensive ingredients for your family to raise healthy, happy eaters. (You'll learn more about why in the chapter on Nutrition.) And your child doesn't *need* to like or even eat those kinds of foods in order to be healthy. (In fact, being overly concerned or trying too hard to change her mind about them can backfire, as you'll learn in Chapter 6 on Trust.)

While I don't recommend you stop yourself from seeking out ideas for healthy eating and family meals from the media, I do recommend you take stock of how and whether their influence is helping—or stressing you out, making you feel defeated, or causing you to judge your or your child's food preferences as not good or healthy enough. We can take a cue from media literacy programs to make sure food parenting influencers aren't impacting us in a negative way by keeping the following questions in mind when we scroll through images of food and snack ideas on social media or thumb through the pages of a beautiful cookbook.

What's This Food Blogger or Cookbook Author's Purpose? Is this Snickerdoodle Cauliflower Breakfast Bar that "your kids will love" created with the purpose of making your life as a parent easier? Or is meant to make the author look clever for sneaking in so many superfoods into one ingredient list? Or is it a sponsored recipe, created with the purpose of getting you to click, click, click or buy a specific brand or ingredient?

Is This Realistic? Identify what about the image, recipe, or family meal plan is so appealing to you. Is it the easy-to-find ingredients and low-stress prep instructions? Or the kids' smiling faces, bright and immaculately clean countertops, or the sleek teak bowl the food is being served in? In other words, things you're not necessarily going to get even if you do decide to cook this way.

Is This Worth It? If you were to take this person's advice and make a whole week's worth of meals from scratch, how much time would it really take you? How much more money would it cost you? And would missing that time with your kids (or for self-care or a passion project) create enough benefits to be worth it?

Appreciate What You're Doing Right. If you start to feel guilty because you're not taking time to mix spinach-based pancakes or blend beet-based breakfast smoothies like that mom on Instagram, remind yourself of the two, three, or ten things you have done already today to make sure your child is cared for and well-fed.

Be Mindful of Emotions. Do a self-check while scrolling, watching videos, or turning the pages of a cookbook. Are you feeling excited, empowered, and inspired or tense, fearful, or pressured? If a food or cooking-related media source isn't serving you well, spend less time consuming it.

INFLUENCE OF PUBERTY

Adolescence and preadolescence are marked by the beginning and progression of puberty. For girls, this developmental stage is marked by changes in body composition, including an increase and redistribution of body fat. Since these normal and developmentally appropriate changes tend to pull a girl's body away from the thin ideal, their body dissatisfaction tends to ratchet up more during these years. At the same time, the hormonal changes and accompanying growth spurt trigger an increase in appetite during puberty. So along with an increase in body fat, girls may be seeking out more food and higher-calorie foods. Thanks to diet culture and internalized weight stigma (aka fatphobia), this creates the perfect storm for young girls to start worrying about their eating. In fact, these changes give at least some insight into why these years are when girls are also at the highest risk for eating disorders.

However, we don't have to get caught up in the storm right alongside them. The more educated we, as parents, are about the normality of these changes in body composition and appetite, the better we are able to make sure they don't similarly ratchet up our own anxiety about our daughter's weight or eating or future health. To be clear, girls tend put on weight in preparation for puberty or before more obvious signs of puberty, such as menstruation, occur. If you see a rounded belly emerge around 9 or 10 years old (or even earlier depending on factors such as race, ethnicity and exposure to stress and adversity) we can reassure ourselves that our daughters' bodies are doing exactly what they are meant to. With our own acceptance in place, we can normalize a changing or fattening up of the body for our daughters too.

If we have a solid IFM in place and we understand how our fears of fat might influence when we notice changes in our daughters' bodies, we will be less likely to feel burdened and concerned about them. And the extra knowledge can give us further reason why we don't want to see, for example, the emergence of some extra belly fat as impetus to consider telling our daughter that her increase in appetite is causing a problem or that she needs to start "eating healthy," which in our current culture is a thinly veiled encouragement to stop gaining weight.

If you're still not convinced that your daughter's body changes or weight increases are keeping in line with what's developmentally normal for her during the pubertal stage, you can use your daughter's growth chart as a point of reference and reassurance. Tracking changes in height, weight, and BMI percentiles over time—and whether they match up to what's expected during different developmental changes—can help you differentiate whether your child's weight really is suddenly going up at a faster-than-normal rate or if it is more a matter of your perception or the influence of diet culture. (Find more information on understanding growth charts and changes in body weight in Chapter 5 or ask a weight-inclusive or HAES®-informed provider to evaluate and interpret them for you.)

INFLUENCE OF HEALTH ASSIGNMENTS, SCHOOL, & TEACHERS

Maybe it's a health assignment asking your daughter to track her daily food and calculate her calories, a weigh-in meant to help the school determine her BMI, or a letter home from her teacher warning you to "please only send in healthy snacks such as fruits and vegetables." Whatever the case, these are all examples of how schools teach parents and children to associate limiting, restricting, and thinness with health and well-being. While I'd love to say we can assume that schools are well aware of the risks of eating disorders and are doing all they can to protect our children from them, judging from the stories I've heard from other mothers and teens, I simply can't. For now, it's up to parents to be proactive and ferret out the kinds of teaching and information that might tip the scales for an already pressured child and cause them to become even more anxious or self-conscious about their eating or their weight.

So how can you fend off negative education-related influences? If you know older parents in your daughter's district, ask if they've had any experience with health assignments (or diet-centric teachers) that ask kids to monitor their eating, exercise, or weight. Call the school's health office and ask if and how they collect children's BMI (it differs state-by-state). Take note if the school is telling you which foods your child "should" and "shouldn't" be bringing in; it's a red flag that they have no problem passing their own food beliefs and judgements along to your daughter. If you need a hand when it comes to confronting administrators, curriculum developers, or teachers about the negative impacts of assignments, policies, or rules, I have good news. We're all in luck! Eating disorder experts who advocate for eradicating harmful messages about food and weight have created a host of compelling, evidence-based letters that address many of the ways diet culture shows up in school. (You can link to resources at nourishher.com/school.)

REFLECTIONS ON INFLUENCE

- *Which influences do you think impact your daughter the most when it comes to her eating or thoughts about dieting? (Friends, family, social media, school, or other, for example.)*

- *In what ways is the source of influence impacting your daughter's eating? In what ways is this influence impacting her thoughts about her body? About dieting? Her health? Or weight or weight loss?*

- *If the influence is harmful, what is one action you could take to lessen its impact on your daughter?*

- *If the influence is positive, what is one way you can increase her exposure to it?*

CHAPTER FOUR
WELL-BEING

"I choose to be happy because it is good for my health."

—*Voltaire*

W HEN JESSICA FIRST PHONED ME TO SET UP AN APPOINTMENT for nutrition therapy, she was like so many other mothers when I meet them for the first time: She was worried about her daughter's health and she was trying to help her lose weight to improve it. At the same time, she was feeling a tremendous amount of conflict, guilt, and shame for her efforts.

Jessica was referred to me through the same pinball labyrinth that many parents raising a child in a larger body bounce through on their way to a pediatric dietitian. It started when she took her daughter, Sarah, in for her 10-year-old well-child visit with her long-time pediatrician. The pediatrician did what many do: She noted that Sarah's BMI percentile had increased since her last visit. Now that Sarah was at the 86th percentile, she fell into a classification that the medical community calls "overweight." Sarah's pediatrician explained to both Sarah and her mother that the change was something to keep an eye on, then suggested she avoid juice, eat more vegetables, and move at least 60 minutes per day.

While hearing the word "overweight" was upsetting to both mom and Sarah, the second aspect of the conversation was even more difficult to process. While Sarah had always been notably larger than her two sisters, she was just as active—if not more so—and was regarded by both her parents as their best eater, enjoying vegetables and fish just as much as she did classic kid foods such as pasta and breads. If she wasn't considered a healthy eater now, when would she be? Mom shared with me in our session that she'd been angry and confused since that visit because, "Sarah *already* eats so healthy."

During the three months between that initial visit with the pediatrician and her first visit with me, a lot had changed between mother and daughter. Since the pediatrician had also noted that Sarah's father had high cholesterol and her maternal grandfather had type 2 diabetes, she referred the family to a pediatric endocrinologist for an additional workup and evaluation.

At the endocrinologist's office, Jessica questioned the bloodwork that was being ordered for Sarah. She was told it was a routine recommendation meant to screen for problems associated with being overweight such as diabetes, heart disease, and high blood pressure. While Sarah's bloodwork turned out to be just fine, Jessica couldn't shake the worry that her daughter's weight wasn't just a point of difference between her and her other daughters, but a potential time bomb that would one day wreak major havoc on Sarah's health if she didn't get it under control.

With those fears in mind, every meal and snack had become an increasing source of stress for this mother of three. She started analyzing her daughter's eating in a way she never had before. Thanks to many years of trying to push her own weight down on the scale, she knew all of the many strategies for losing—and maintaining—a smaller physique. Everything Sarah ate was now being scanned by the calorie calculator that Jessica had in her brain, which she had worked hard to put to sleep in herself over a decade ago. Carbs and fats were also potential problems she saw in every meal; a smear of butter on her morning toast, a slice of cheddar on the sandwiches she packed for lunch, a scoop of ice cream on a sunny afternoon. Jessica couldn't help but sink deeper into worry and wonder about whether it was too much with every bite her daughter enjoyed.

To make it worse, Sarah was smart, sensitive, and a bit of a perfectionist, qualities that her mother knew made her daughter vulnerable to anxiety. So while Jessica was dead set on bringing her daughter's BMI back down and cutting out the disease-causing culprits, she was wracking her brain about how she might do it without tripping her daughter's own worry into overdrive. Every change she made to meals, she did as covertly as she could with the specific intention of protecting her daughter's mental health and self-esteem.

Despite mom being careful to avoid overtly and explicitly limiting her daughter's food, Sarah had gotten the message that her eating was an issue. The family meals mom and dad prepared now included twice as many vegetables and little if any of the carbohydrates they once enjoyed, including her mom's beloved sweet potato fries. Her father and sisters seemed stressed. Mom was spending hours planning out "healthy" meals, insisting on trying dishes they'd never heard of, nixed desserts completely, and was packing things in their lunches that they'd considered foreign, tasteless, and bland. Worse, Sarah felt responsible. While she'd noticed her weight had been changing, being labeled with the "o" word made her feel ashamed of her body in a way she'd never felt before. She had vowed to fix things by putting herself on a diet, throwing out half or more of her lunch and giving away her after-school snacks to some of the younger girls at soccer and dance practice.

By the time this mother and daughter came into my office, they were feeling frustrated, unhappy, insecure, and confused about eating *and* Sarah's health. While the pediatrician and endocrinologist visits were made with the intention of helping Sarah, from what I could tell the outcome had been just the opposite. The conversations about changing BMI, the term "overweight" and its potentially dire-sounding consequences, the increased shame both mom and daughter now felt about Sarah's weight, and the heightened mealtime stress and uncertainty about eating were taking significant tolls on both mother and daughter individually, as well as on their shared relationship and connection.

GOOD HEALTH VERSUS WELL-BEING

Jessica's desire to protect her daughter's physical health is a universal one. We put physical health on a pedestal, attribute virtue, morals and values to it, and consider it to be an unequivocal desire. We don't question the sometimes bizarre or extraordinary steps people take to pursue avoiding disease and getting their bodies into tip-top shape. And we don't question others—doctors, dietitians, media outlets, cultural standards, pseudo-scientists, book authors, etc.—when they press an agenda of achieving optimal physical health upon us.

As parents, we are more than willing to go to bat with our kids in challenging ways to protect their health on a daily—if not hourly—basis. We battle with them to get to sleep on time and we negotiate with them (and then berate and question ourselves about the terms we agree to) when it comes to the amount of technology they're exposed to. We wrestle with them to apply and reapply sufficient amounts of sunscreen and bug spray after studying the labels to avoid overexposing them to harmful chemicals, we inspect their teeth to make sure they're brushing correctly, and we check and recheck (in sometimes embarrassing ways) to make sure they're moving their bowels in normal and consistent ways. It only makes sense that we would intervene in an issue as integral to their health as their eating, too. The ways in which we do it, the benefits and harms, and our overall objectives are something I believe we have to look deeper into, however, if we truly want to do right by our children.

As a pediatric nutritionist, I have been forced to reckon with the ways we intervene with behaviors, habits, and preferences for food. After suffering so much by diligently focusing on my own eating and monitoring my weight, for example, how could I possibly recommend to other parents, such as Jessica, that she teach Sarah to do the same? On the other hand, I was trained as a public health professional to regard pediatric obesity as a national epidemic. If I wanted to support parents in raising healthier eaters, wasn't teaching them how to reverse their child's weight gain a major part of the equation? If so, then why did conversations around those topics feel shameful, destructive, and potentially harmful instead of feeling positive, beneficial, and therapeutic?

For the first four years of my career, I worked in a major New York pediatric endocrinology practice, which meant the majority of my patients were children at the highest risks for diseases and dysfunctions commonly thought to be caused by their elevated body weight. I confronted this internal struggle constantly. I was faced with recommending the clinical and traditional approaches—all of which revolved around weight loss and management—for treating problems such as type 2 diabetes, insulin resistance, and elevated cholesterol and triglycerides. Sarah was just one of dozens of girls—hundreds of adolescents—who felt self-conscious, insecure, and unsure about her body, weight, food choices, and her physical activity. And she, like others, seemed in danger of approaching that same precipice of dieting and disordered eating that I had tread on myself.

To resolve my internal conflict, I had to start thinking more deeply about what we as parents and healthcare providers mean when we talk about good health and healthy eating.

Good health, as it turns out, is about much more than avoiding diabetes, cardiovascular disease, and metabolic dysfunction. It's about more than getting adequate sleep and protecting our kids from cancer, West Nile virus, tooth decay, and constipation. And when it came to Sarah and girls like her, protecting her health was not about helping her get below the 86th BMI percentile.

Good health is broader and more all-encompassing than any of those things. According to the World Health Organization (WHO), "Health is a state of complete physical, mental and social well-being, and not merely the absence of disease or infirmity."[1] To make peace with my conflicts about how to support children struggling with weight changes in the most humane, positive, and effective way possible, I started holding this holistic definition of health in mind whenever a challenging question arose. It assuaged the public health advocate in me as sound advice, it reassured the mother in me as an empathetic approach, and it felt worthy and protective for the vulnerable and intelligent young girls I was working with. Eventually, it started guiding my approach to everything about nutrition and eating.

As such, for the majority of my clients I stopped focusing on healthy eating, which traditionally centered on eating as a way to support and protect physical health, and which often includes lowering body weight; but as far as I could tell, it had the side-effects of triggering a host of other issues related to disordered and chaotic eating. Instead, I changed my approach to nutrition to be one that had a much larger, more holistic view, one that would protect my patients' and clients'—even my own daughters'—well-being.

I started thinking about approaches to eating that supported physical health and the avoidance of disease as equally as they support us emotionally and socially. In my practice and in my home, when I talked about and aimed for healthy eating, what I was really hoping to achieve was *eating well-being*.

WHAT IS EATING WELL-BEING?

When I use the term *eating well-being*, I mean eating in ways that support our physical health, emotional health, and relationships equally. Unlike current notions of "healthy eating," it avoids promoting eating habits, styles, attitudes, and behaviors that focus on improving physical health at the expense of making us feel ashamed or stressed, pressuring us to choose foods and cooking methods that are unpleasant or unfamiliar, thwarting our ability to be social creatures, or threatening relationships with those we love. When we focus on eating well-being, we allow ourselves to eat in ways that are pleasant and enjoyable, and that support us holistically instead.

In the case of Sarah, for example, the goal of health was one that her mother, pediatrician, and I shared. Yet our notions of what "healthy" meant differed greatly—and so do our approaches.

From the pediatrician's perspective, physical health was at the forefront; according to an algorithm she was likely using to determine what steps to take with her patient, getting the BMI percentile back down below the 86th percentile was the goal, ordering blood work to screen for related diseases was the approach she would use to meet it, and alerting her caregiver of the percentile meaning and change was her way of doing it.

Sarah's mom was juggling concerns about physical and emotional health, both wanting her daughter's BMI to go down and also wanting to protect her from the stress and shame of worrying about her weight and dieting. Unfortunately, Sarah was already feeling the indignity and guilt that is so often brought on when a young woman has their body size identified as a problem needing to be fixed. And without a model for a positive way to approach their concern, mother and daughter's way of relating to one another around family meals and communicating about food became stressed and uncertain.

After hearing a little bit about Sarah's story, I saw clearly how she was suffering emotionally—and how she and her mother seemed fractured in relation to one another. In speaking with her privately, I also learned that she'd been throwing out her after-school snacks and skipping lunch without her mother knowing. With this in mind, I was concerned that her physical health was now at risk, too.

My approach for supporting this mother and daughter is the same one I recommend for so many of my clients, which is to reexamine what each of them individually and then collectively mean when they talk about the goal of being a "healthy eater." When those ideals are limited or restrictive, even punitive, I explain the concept of *eating well-being* and suggest they deliberately aim for this more holistic goal instead.

PROTECTING WELL-BEING

When it came to helping Sarah, I believe taking her overall well-being into account would have made all the difference.

First, instead of overtly flagging the change on her growth chart and emphasizing the classification of the BMI percentiles, her pediatrician could have discussed the body weight change privately with her mother, as opposed to sharing them with her in front of her 10-year-old. In fact, avoiding talking about weight directly with a child has been suggested to pediatricians in a paper published by the American Academy of Pediatrics—a fact that I think all parents need to know about.

Second, the provider could have gone a step further and, instead of trying to correct or "treat" her weight, she could have explained to mom the importance of avoiding *focusing* on Sarah's weight at all, as well as the importance of avoiding weight loss. Additionally, to protect Sarah from possible harm, she could have also explained that she was making these recommendations based on the fact that adolescents who start diets in an attempt to lose weight are at an increased risk for, ironically, weight gain and binge eating. And worse, they're more likely to develop an eating disorder.[2] If she'd had a few extra seconds, she could have added the importance of parents avoiding talking about their own weight and dieting in front of their children.

As a parent with a history of disordered eating and a pediatric dietitian who confronts negative food and dieting-related beliefs in parents all the time, I believe it would be extremely worthwhile if pediatricians take additional steps and—before they make recommendations for exactly how best to address weight changes—ask a parent about their own history with food, dieting, and weight changes. *Have you ever had an eating disorder? Do you engage in dieting? Have you ever felt stressed about what to eat or felt overly concerned about managing your weight? Have you ever engaged in restrictive or extreme weight loss diets?* A tendency toward disordered eating can be passed down through generations, making children of parents with unhealthy relationships with food more vulnerable to developing them.[3] If a parent has struggled with food in the past, it's important to identify that risk factor just like they would any other, be it diabetes or heart disease. In an ideal world, identifying this risk factor would be an opportunity to offer resources for extra support for parenting around food just like they would offer a referral to an endocrinologist or other specialist.

Finally, focusing on eating well-being—as opposed to eating to reduce body weight—could help protect Sarah from an eating dysfunction that could ultimately wreak havoc on her physical health, smash her self-esteem, fracture her relationship with her mother, and create stress with the rest of the family. As a nutrition counselor, that's the approach I took. Instead of ramping up vigilance against weight gain by micromanaging intake, I did just the opposite: I helped mom and daughter have a more positive and relaxed attitude toward specific foods, food groups, and macro and micronutrients. By letting go of the ideas of healthy eating that they had in their minds, which included limiting and restricting, calorie counting, and vegetable loading, Sarah was able to give herself permission to start eating lunch again. This was a great step towards turning away from disorder and rebuilding her own eating competence.

The change also restored some equilibrium to the family's eating dynamics, making meals more relaxed, fun, and connective experiences. Creating an open and positive dialogue about what good eating could look like for them also helped to mend Sarah and Jessica's relationship. In time, these changes improved Sarah's overall physical and emotional health as well. With increased eating competence, Sarah has been much better protected from disordered eating, as well as much closer to restoring her original BMI percentile, improving her overall nutrient intake, and increasing her self-esteem. She and her mom have also enjoyed more ease at the table, with both enjoying a wider variety of foods, and Jessica often comments in our sessions that her daughter seems "less on edge" and "happier" at dinner and that she herself has been "relieved" to no longer feel like she has to manage her daughter's eating.

To be clear, significant changes in BMI percentile are an important part of assessing a child's overall health. However, addressing those changes in a more nuanced way can have a profound impact on a child's overall well-being and lifelong relationship with food. When pediatricians and parents note and address these changes with a child's overall well-being in mind, they can avoid triggering eating dysfunction and the unhealthy shifts in BMI that are linked with dieting.

Luckily, it was something her mother instinctively felt ambivalent about. And while she wanted to take doctor's orders, she tried her best to do it in a way that did as little harm as possible. She naturally tried to protect her daughter's well-being, but without insight and "permission" from a health professional to avoid focusing on reversing that BMI percentile, she felt confused, overwhelmed, and conflicted by it.

The majority of pediatricians are on extreme time constraints and, unless they are particularly sensitive to eating dysfunction and weight issues or have experience with eating disorders, there's a chance that they might not have the time or the knowledge to address changes to BMI in a sensitive, holistic way.

With that in mind, we can protect our daughters—all our children, in fact—against inadvertent pressure to diet that might come along with a medical visit. If you suspect your pediatrician might bring up weight or weight changes in front of your child, you can find tips to protect her before her next medical visit on page 71.

SKEPTICISM ABOUT EATING WELL-BEING

Allow me to preemptively address any suspicions that might crop up for you or your parenting partners. You see, from my experience, the concept of overall well-being is an easy one for most of us to digest. (Sorry! It's too perfect.) The notion that our child's self-esteem, emotional life, and social connections are just as important to her health as her cholesterol or blood sugar control makes sense. And yet, when I take that notion one step further and suggest we can apply it to our eating, such as eating well-being, parents start to feel uncomfortable.

Eating to support emotional health? "Isn't emotional eating bad for you?" they'll ask. "My son eats because of his anxiety all the time and it's really a problem! You can't be serious." And what could eating for social health mean anyway? "I read that we eat *more* when we're out with friends," says another. "My teenager doesn't make the best choices when she's out with her friends." Since I know from experience questions will come up, let's go a little deeper. What does it really mean to eat in ways that support our emotional, social, and physical health?

EATING FOR EMOTIONAL WELL-BEING

In a book that seeks to help mothers quell worry about their child's eating habits and weight, the topic of emotional eating could take up an entire chapter, maybe two. Right up there with sugar and dessert, emotional eating is one of the topics parents ask me about the most. Often, I hear things from parents like, "She eats because of her anxiety." And then I usually hear, in a hushed tone tinged with guilt that "It's something I struggle with, too." Shame around the notion that we might link our emotions to food abounds. Yet eating is intrinsically an emotional experience. It involves memories and associations, traditions, is often done together with loved ones, and let's not underestimate the fact that it's a life-sustaining act! It makes sense that eating would trigger positive feelings such as joy, reassurance, and comfort. Unfortunately, eating can be even more emotional when we approach food with efforts and intentions like weight loss or control. Negative feelings, such as guilt and remorse, get stirred up when we enjoy foods or eat amounts we think we shouldn't, which colors the emotional landscape at the table even more.

I can't pinpoint exactly when it was determined that emotional eating is a habit that needs to be fixed, but I'm pretty sure it started with someone highlighting research linking it to weight gain. That's probably one reason that diet culture then made the resolute promise that in order to reclaim our thinner, healthier selves we needed to divest ourselves of emotions at meals. Regardless of how emotional eating gained such a profound stigma, one way I've been able to help unravel the harm of it is to point out to parents the necessity of *linking* emotions with eating. After that, we can have an easier time deciding how best to—or whether we even should—address emotional eating in ourselves and our kids.

First, doesn't it make perfect sense that every activity we must engage in to be alive should be an enjoyable one? Eating is an act of self-sustenance, the ultimate act of self-care. Without joy and positive emotions associated with it, how will we ever be driven to do it? (Yes, there's an obvious analogy. I encourage you to think about it! And I *also* encourage you to avoid taking it for granted. For some, eating is a joyless or even terrifying act. For example, people who have feeding tubes, have lost the ability to taste, chew or swallow solids, are in recovery from eating disorders, or who have had significant physical or emotional trauma with food can find eating a mechanical process or arduous challenge.) Since we need to eat daily, multiple times a day in fact, it only makes sense that, biologically speaking, the act is done best when it is a pleasurable one and it helps if we respect or even feel grateful for our ability to enjoy it.

Eating is not just physically fulfilling; it can bring relief, it can soothe. Even in its simplest form, eating can calm us. Think about our infant child's experience, the emotions she felt with hunger and satiety, both obvious and extreme. When hunger started to build, she felt at first uncomfortable, then increasingly irritable. If that hunger went un-addressed too long, she cried that special high-alert infant cry that—to this day—makes everyone's emotions rattle. (Just thinking about my littlest crying out in hunger fills me with panic, concern, and—brace yourself for some TMI—makes my boobs tingle a bit. And as soon as she was fed, she and I were both calm and soothed.)

It's often suggested that positive emotions are meant to be tied to eating for good reason. The more joy we get out of eating, the better we will be. I know that flies right in the face of diet culture, which has us thinking, "Yeah, but *too much* joy in eating is dangerous, isn't it?" Nope. Just the opposite, in fact; finding joy in eating has a function and is protective.

When we take pleasure in something, when we enjoy it, we are more willing to put more creative effort into doing it. If eating were purely a rote function, like brushing our teeth, then I doubt we'd be as willing and interested in investing time, energy, and other countless resources to keep attending to it in new and exciting ways. If there were not so much gustatory joy to be had in eating, I'm pretty sure I'd swallow down the same exact meal morning, noon, and night without much thought, effort, or deviation, just like I've been slathering on the same dollop more or less of fluoride-fortified paste on my teeth for the past fifteen years.

Enjoying a variety of foods has long been a hallmark of good nutritional health, however, so we must be inspired to seek out many different foods and opportunities to eat day after day, meal after meal. Getting joy, pleasure, and physical delight in food is a beautiful way our biology inspires us to do it. In fact, people who lose their sense of smell and taste often lose their pleasure in eating, not to mention their interest in changing up the menu every few meals or reaching for a forkful of something new from what's on their plate. Thus, their nutritional status plummets, too. We don't need to fear the pleasure and satisfaction we take in eating a piece of chocolate ganache as if it were as detrimental to our health, such as a love for inhaling the tobacco in a cigarette. Pleasure, joy, and reward work in our favor and are all part of the grand scheme to keep us nourished and well.

With all this in mind, it makes sense that at times when we are stressed, depressed, anxious, or isolated, we might seek out food as a salve, a comfort, and an emotional healer. We can get instant and temporary relief from enjoying the same homemade ravioli that our mother always made on Sunday nights, the heavily frosted store-bought cake our uncle always brought to Thanksgiving, and the dumplings our bestie always picks up for us when we are feeling sick or down.

Here's what we as parents (and emotional eaters, if we identify this way ourselves) need to pay attention to. Emotional eating does have its purpose and strengths. Pleasurable foods are usually easy to access and the relief they provide from uncomfortable emotions is instant. Carbohydrates—or glucose—are the main energy source for every cell in our body and our brains know that our bodies need this nutrient to survive. Thus, we get an immediate and powerful neurological reward when we eat it, particularly if it's an easily digestible and quickly absorbed form, such as sugar. That reward comes in the form of dopamine, a brain chemical that boosts mood and makes us feel good. We're not bad or unhealthy because we tend to crave sugary foods when we're down; in my mind, we're just the opposite. Our bodies are listening to and responding to our mood (and even our blood sugar level, if we haven't eaten for a while or eaten enough) and are very intelligently and protectively driving us to look for an effective way to correct it.

Likewise, fat is also neurologically rewarding, perhaps because each gram contains more than twice as many calories as other nutrients such as carbohydrates and proteins. Despite our current cultural belief that calories are something to be feared and avoided, our bodies know that they're valuable and needed to survive. Since our mouths can literally sense the presence of this particularly good energy source, it makes sense that we'd be primed to feel reassured by, and get pleasure from, eating foods that contain it.[4] And it also makes sense that a Krispy Creme donut—which contains both sugar and fat—be the source of even more neurobiological reward and delight!

That understood, emotional eating also has a weakness and a rub. First, the mood boost we get is only temporary and at surface level. It doesn't fix the underlying issue we are struggling with. If we use food to get a mood boost or comfort without *also* resolving what's troubling us, we are going to run into some problems, particularly if it's an ongoing or long-term issue. Second, if we feel conflicted about enjoying those comforting foods, thanks to our internalized attitudes that they are "taboo," any emotional relief will be followed by worsening of our stress, anxiety, or otherwise negative mood since it's now been doused with guilt, shame, and remorse.

To help our daughters get the soothing benefits of food that support their well-being *without* the subsequent harm, we need to first do our best to decipher if her emotional eating is positive and occasional, or negative and chronic. If your daughter uses food to soothe occasionally while also acknowledging the underlying stressor, then we do best by helping her get a truly therapeutic mood boost untainted by feelings of guilt and shame. Our work is to help neutralize any negative feelings she—and you—may have towards the foods she enjoys and finds soothing but may feel conflicted about.

For example, if your daughter wants to stop for frozen yogurt after finding out she failed an algebra test she spent a lot of time studying for, that could be positive and soothing. The warm fuzzies she gets from eating a food she normally associated with better times makes sense. Plus, enjoying it with her would be a great time to acknowledge her disappointment as well as talk about a plan to get her some more math help. I consider that a positive example of emotional eating that we can ignore and a type of self-care we can even feel good about. If eating enjoyable foods does cause her or you lots of guilt or shame, you use the information in Chapter 4 to help neutralize unnecessarily negative feelings about certain foods. If she doesn't feel an aftermath of negative emotions about doing it, even better. If you can just accept it for what it is without judgment—dare I suggest to even take some pride in the fact that she's actively seeking powerful and instant relief from emotional pain—then your work is done!

If, on the other hand, you notice that your daughter is picking up the same yogurt every day after school, despite the fact that she's not hungry or is indulging in another comforting food frequently in a way that's isolating and habitual, she may be doing so to avoid long-term and uncomfortable underlying emotions, such as depression, boredom, loneliness, low self-esteem, or poor peer relationships. This behavior would be negative and chronic in my mind. If you suspect that your daughter is frequently eating as a way to soothe difficult emotions, she may be doing what I call *evasive eating*.

When we repeatedly seek temporary relief from emotional discomfort without addressing the source of that pain, we miss out on an opportunity to resolve it. In addition, we very often create additional problems. If our child is struggling to handle a move, a new school, or a loss of a relationship with *evasive eating*, we need to intervene—but not on the eating itself. *Evasive eating* may artificially inflate or destabilize our weight, which can ultimately harm our physical and social well-being in unnecessary ways. However, while sudden weight gain or a potential worsening of diet-related conditions might feel like the primary concern, I believe there's a much more worthwhile and beneficial approach that we can focus on. *Evasive eating* can be a signal that our daughters are hurting and lacking other more effective, everlasting, and powerful coping mechanisms for dealing with it. Instead of focusing on curbing emotional eating, we can do better by doing the harder work of focusing on helping our daughters build a toolbox of skills she can rely on when processing uncomfortable emotions—or whatever is at the root of her emotional pain.

A psychotherapist is best positioned to help your daughter build up this toolbox. Skills in her toolbox might include building more positive interpersonal relationships, such as peer friendships, getting enough sleep, utilizing mindfulness, taking part in regular, enjoyable physical movement, talking more frequently with a trusted adult such as a school counselor, social worker, or psychologist, or even doing emotion-focused writing or journaling.[5]

The truth is, children who are doing *evasive eating* need support with emotions, not healthy eating recommendations. And the more we can remember this, the better able we will be to help our daughters and avoid damaging their relationship to food and feelings about their body even more.

There is no "cure" for emotional or evasive eating, but there is the knowledge that it is in some ways very natural and can signal that we or our daughters need something more. Some evidence suggests that, thanks to genetic traits, some of us are more prone to using food to self-regulate or soothe negative or uncomfortable emotions, thanks to the fact that they get a bigger dopamine boost—i.e., a bigger emotional reward—when eating sugary, high-calorie foods.[6] Of course, we don't know which type of genes our child has, nor do we necessarily want to know. (I can only imagine how complicated and uncomfortable enjoying an ice cream cone together might be with *that* knowledge in hand!) Simply knowing that there's a *possibility* that any one of us might be more prone to over rely on foods for emotional support can help us be aware of and on alert for a tendency to regularly, and primarily. cope with stress with food.

• •

TIPS FOR PROTECTING AGAINST EVASIVE EATING

A few ways we can be extra protective against *evasive eating* in our daughters and ourselves include:

- *Avoid Dieting.* Research suggests that the more you restrict your child, the higher the chances your child will go overboard on certain foods when a negative emotion or stress strikes. This is especially important to think about if you're a parent who has been trying to limit foods for fear of weight gain—the more your child is feeling stressed about her eating weight or how you and others regard her eating or weight, the more likely she might binge on food.

- *Challenge Your Food Attitudes.* When you feel more relaxed and less concerned, worried, or guilty about enjoying foods, you're less likely to feel the double-jeopardy of emotional eating. In other words, if you do enjoy a bowl of creamy cheddar cheese soup from your favorite homestyle restaurant to take the edge off a stressful afternoon, feeling more positive about food and less worried can support your ability to avoid guilt afterwards. If you can neutralize the negative attitudes you and she have towards these taboo yet comforting foods, she *can* enjoy them without extra conflict. (You can learn more about providing this support in the Chapters on Acceptance and Nutrition.)

- *Learn the Real Meaning of Sneaking.* If you've discovered that your daughter has been sneaking food after school at a friend's home or in her bedroom, consider that it may be a sign that she's feeling too controlled with food either in the types or the amounts she's allowed to eat. Most parents' instinct is to tighten the reins around food even more. Instead, I challenge you to take an alternative action that will serve your daughter even better in the long run. Since sneaking food can often be a sign a child feels ashamed about eating it, use the behavior as an impetus to start making whatever she's been eating in secret more available and part of a regular routine. If it's potato or tortilla chips, for example, you might consider offering some in place of another starchy food, such as roast potatoes or a bowl of corn. Cookies or candy can be offered as a dessert or alongside some fruit and cheese as a snack. Giving her an opportunity to eat forbidden foods out in the open and without shame, guilt, or limits can help her feel calmer and more in control when enjoying them. Doing so lessens internal conflict and increases calmness and joy. With those positive emotions in place, it will be easier for her to listen to her body and find her natural stopping point—something that is nearly impossible to do when you're rushing to finish and hide the evidence before you're found out. It will also help her enjoy these foods in a balanced way as she has more access to them in years to come.

- *Help Her Name Emotions.* Pay close attention to how well she is able to identify what she's feeling. Even if she's indulging in a food for comfort, can she talk about what's bothering her? Or is it as deeply buried as those chocolate bar wrappers under her bed? Children who are able to label emotions cope better, are more resilient, have more stable and positive relationships, have a positive self-im-age, do better in school, and have fewer behavior issues.[7] (To access an emotions wheel, which can make it easier for your daughter to identify and talk about some of what she's feeling, visit NourishHer.com/feelings.)

Remember, these tips aren't meant to be used as a way to stop you or your daughter from emotional eating, which can get complicated and start to feel like another type of restriction, diet, or weight control method. Nor are they meant as a way to process difficult feelings, which can be challenging without the help of a professional. Rather, they are meant to start increasing awareness of our feelings without judgement.

It's important to note that emotional eating isn't yet well under-stood, nor is it the same experience for everyone. Since this book is dedicated to protecting our daughters from diet culture, I chose to address how those of us who have been primarily taught to regard emo-tional eating—with a fear of weight gain. However, emotions might impact our children's eating in endless other ways.

The idea, for example, that food is comforting and reassuring isn't true for everyone. Some children *avoid* eating when they are feeling scared or anxious. Feeling anxious might be part of their temperament or be situational if there's a lot of conflict at the table, be it about the food itself or other family circumstances or relationships. Some children have negative emotions triggered by food because of past trauma such as a feeding difficulty, a severe allergy, gastrointestinal experience such as food poisoning, forced feeding, or other reasons. Some kids might have a set of negative emotions linked with food due to chronic food in-security if, for example, they haven't had the privilege of having access to enough food or not having access to enough food consistently. (Note that food insecurity could be a literal absence of food or a psychological deprivation, say if a parent themselves are withholding food due worries about weight gain, a food allergy, blood sugar control, or other reasons.)

If you're parenting multiple types of children—like one who is overly excited by and focused on food or uses it to soothe, and another who is indifferent or would avoid eating completely if you allowed her to—don't fret. I have had many parents supporting children on both sides of the eating spectrum. Ultimately, I encourage you to use this fact as proof that every child has a unique eating history, temperament, and emotional and physical response to food. While you as a mother are here to support them as best you can, be reassured that you are neither responsible for nor in control of those aspects of their eating.

EATING FOR SOCIAL WELL-BEING

Just like a ginormous holiday dinner with your closest friends and family, eating for social health has both a bright side and a dark side.

To start, we are *meant* to eat together. Evolutionarily speaking, we could survive much longer and in better ways if we shared our resources. So, it makes sense that, in general, families who eat together would get a primal and powerful biochemical reinforcement. Eating with others has been shown to help you work better together as a team. Eating the same foods seems to reinforce positive vibes even more, promoting a special kind of bonding that's linked to an increased willingness to be cooperative and an ability to come to agreements more quickly.[8] All that shared, face-to-face contact likely improves our communication skills. Perhaps that's why families who eat together tend to function better as a unit and individually.[9] Children and adolescents who regularly eat with their family have more stable body weights, lower rates of cardiovascular disease, and an increased intake of fruits and vegetables and nutrients such as calcium. Not surprisingly, their mental health gets a boost, too. They have better peer relationships, lower rates of anxiety, depression, and eating disorders, and are less likely to participate in risky behaviors. They also do better academically, have a larger vocabulary, and experience increased protection against cyberbullying.[10]

Even with all of the benefits in mind, packed schedules and long working hours can make eating meals together as a family still feel out of reach. One way to make family meals easier? Stop worrying about how healthy or unhealthy the foods you serve are and whether your kids did or didn't eat their vegetables. Research shows your kids get all the benefits of family meals *regardless* of what is being served and eaten. Turns out, it's simply the act of being together—the social aspect—during eating that matters most. To help you and your daughter get the benefits, stress less about what's on the table and focus your energy on listening and connecting instead. One thing that the moms I work with and I like to remember during family meals—Eyes up! If you find your mind drifting back to taking inventory of how much or little your child has eaten, make it a point to pull your eyes up off their plate and focus on their faces instead.

In addition to increasing our feelings of connection, some evidence suggests that our eating habits improve when we do it in a social way, as opposed to eating alone.[11] While you might feel like things were easier when you only had to worry about feeding yourself instead of multiple people, eating alone wasn't necessarily doing you any good.

If you've ever been single, you might have noticed that cooking for a party of one can sometimes feel, well, like it's not worth all the trouble. Sure, as a mother I regularly fantasize about all spider rolls, saag paneer, and spicy peanut tofu bowls I'd prefer to eat for dinner, but the sad truth is that when I lived alone and had just myself to feed, I was more inclined to quickly scrounge for some questionable, still-safe-to-eat-leftovers, eat quickly while standing in front of the fridge, leave out multiple food groups, get by with some popcorn and few slices of cheese or a bowl of ice cream, or skip a meal altogether. Once I started eating with an audience night after night—and even when it was just my husband—I became a much better eater in the sense that meals contained multiple edible food groups, differed from night to night, were eaten at a table while sitting, and with actual utensils as opposed to straight from the package with my fingers.

In fact, I've noticed in my own life that the more people I have to cook for and eat with, the more elaborate the meal typically gets—and the more foods I actually eat. And I think you might agree. Compare for a moment what you might prepare when eating by yourself versus what you or your partner might prepare if you were to eat together, versus what you might prepare for a group of company. The more people you are feeding, the more variety goes into planning, which results in more food groups and more nutrients being eaten, right?

In addition to the idea that eating with others tends to make us more accountable for actually feeding ourselves more elaborately and faithfully (and with more dignity, respect, and regard for actual taste and potential food-poisoning), there's also another benefit that simply being with others confers on our emotional well-being. Eating with others is linked with a feeling of being happier and more satisfied with our lives.[12]

So, what's the more sinister side of social eating? Surprise! I'm not going to share the diet culture rhetoric about how eating out at restaurants with friends is bad for your health because of the calories, sodium, or fat the food might contain. Or that talking with friends while eating might—gasp!—cause you to order dessert or eat more than you normally would. Frankly, if you have the time, money, and other resources needed to be able to do this on occasion, feel gratitude for the opportunity and do your best to enjoy it! The dark and disturbing phenomenon that I want to draw your attention to is the fact that in our culture, *not eating* is promoted as a way to improve your social health.

Thanks to weight stigma, not eating promises to give you a whole host of social privilege associated with thinness. However, when we overemphasize a desire to fit in and to be accepted by cultural norms or a desire for thinness, this wreaks havoc on us physically and emotionally. Not eating specific foods or food groups or eating too little of an amount can lead to both macro and micronutrient deficiencies, which can cause irreversible damage to bone and heart health, as well as compromise our neurobiology and, in the case of children, adolescents, and teens, it can stunt bone and organ growth. Not eating enough or frequently enough also makes us irritable, anxious, and distracted.

Ironically, while we might be restricting foods to be thinner and fit in more socially, limiting our diet in rigorous ways can also be extremely stressful on our social lives and relationships. Eating is a social event; therefore, not eating limits social opportunities and can strain close relationships, particularly if they traditionally involve shared meals—for example, in the case of a child eating with her family. If you've ever tried not eating or eating less than you're hungry for, you might remember avoiding certain social situations, such as parties or dinners out with friends as a strategy to minimize the temptation of enjoying the high-calorie food associated with them. I'll admit to skipping a few Super Bowl parties because I was afraid of the endless array of tempting food options such as nachos, wings, cheesy dips, and guac and chips.

The truth is, eating with others improves our emotional well-being and can even improve our eating, while eating in ways that might help you or your daughter fit into a social norm or idealized weight is harmful.

EATING FOR PHYSICAL WELL-BEING

You may not realize it, but most of the news articles, new studies, documentaries, wellness bestsellers, medical doctors, and social media opinions prioritize eating for disease prevention. While that is an admirable goal and, of course, should be considered, many parents will be surprised to learn that a growing number of healthcare providers (particularly nutritionists and mental health experts) filter their ideas about eating through two additional lenses. Learning these alternative views about eating (mentioned earlier in this chapter) can help you feel more objective, relaxed, and confident about your daughter's eating when the "food police" show up in your mind (in the form of a new study or news report) or literally at your dinner table (in the form of dieters, health fanatics, and voracious consumers of wellness best sellers and documentaries). To avoid falling in the trap of overprioritizing disease prevention at the expense of other aspects of eating well-being, keep the following three principals in mind.

First, regardless of what health concern your daughter is being treated for, there is one nutritional concern your dietitian will hold in tandem with—or even prioritize over—all others when they are making eating or feeding recommendations. That principal concern is whether or not she is getting enough nutrition to *support her physical growth*. Even when other health issues—even ones as serious as pre-diabetes, diabetes, insulin resistance, food allergies, celiac disease, ADHD, thyroid disorder or sudden, rapid and unexplained weight gain—are on the table, any dietary changes being made should not be done at the expense of shortchanging our children's bodies of much-needed overall calories and nutrient variety.

Even if your daughter has passed the age of puberty and is no longer growing in height, her bones are still growing in density and strength. Some of her organs, including her brain and lungs, are still growing, too. Thus, protecting against a shortfall of overall calories, macronutrients (such as carbohydrates, fats, and proteins), and micronutrients (such as vitamins and minerals) are essential in order to avoid stunting, delaying, or otherwise compromising her growth even beyond the time when she *look*s like she's "all grown up." It probably goes without saying, but the significant dangers of shortchanging a child on much-needed calories and various nutrients is enough to warrant the avoidance of any type of calorie restricting. (For a shareable list of evidence-based reasons that dieting is harmful for your daughter, visit nourishher.com/9-reasons)

To best support a child's physical growth, we do best to focus on the basics of being well nourished. First and foremost, we want to make sure our child has access to *enough* food, then enough food *consistently*, and then a *variety* of enough food consistently. Once those basic tenets are met, we want to offer food in *a positive and non-judgmental environment* so that she can build her eating competence.

In other words, simply making sure your daughter has access to food in a regular and consistent way and is being fed in an environment that is trusting and accepting of her eating, is the best way to support her physical health, to help her grow, and to help her eat in a way that will lower her risk of both physical diseases and eating disorders. Even if your daughter has certain health concerns, such as high blood pressure or insulin resistance, having these basics in place is essential. Growth is still a primary goal and having a positive, trusting relationship with food sets the stage best for those who want or need to pay special attention to which foods they may need to eat or avoid in the future. Without consistently knowing you'll have enough to eat, you cannot eat well, and children cannot self-regulate nor easily accept new foods or the variety of foods needed to get all the necessary nutrients. You will learn more about the reasons why in further chapters, and I have provided a tool to help you build this consistency. You will also learn more specifics about nutrition. In the meantime, it is important to think about these basic needs—and how much work you are already doing by tending to those needs.

Second, eating and health are infinitely complex topics; registered dietitians know that despite what media headlines claim, no one food or eating habit accounts for disease risk. Diet is only one part of the larger picture of your child's physical health. In my experience, the extent to which most of my clients worry about—and teach their children to fear—foods, nutrients, and ingredients such as sugar, sodium, food dyes, processed foods, fast foods, and GMOs is disproportionate to any physical health benefit one might get by avoiding them. For example, when parents I work with are raising otherwise healthy children and they start trying to keep the diet "clean" to account for every possible health implication, it often ends up harming their child's overall relationship with food by introducing fear, limitations, and restrictions. They either get a rebellious, unhappy, and unwilling eater or an eater who is paralyzed with anxiety about eating the "wrong" or "unhealthy" foods. Worse, parents who are overly focused on the lack of certain health qualities a food has, get distracted from ensuring their child is eating enough food and enough variety to support their growth and relationship with food.

I am not recommending we throw caution to wind and write off eating as a non-important part of health. Far from it! (I have dedicated my entire career to understanding and helping others with matters related to nutrition.) What I *am* saying is that we need to be mindful and intentional about the *areas* of eating that we put our focus on, as well as have realistic expectations and understanding about the importance diet quality and specific foods play on our physical health. I'm saying that we must do our best to avoid giving in to the temptation to worry about the "toxic" nature of added sugar and sodium, processed or fast foods, and refined carbohydrates and over emphasizing the benefits of fruits and vegetables so much that our children end up eating much less of everything altogether. We must remember eating and health are complex, and that no one habit or food defines our health as much as our access to food and our relationship with food.

The third principal that can help you keep a cool head when you feel compelled to worry about how food might impact your daughter's physical health is to be skeptical and analytical about research, and take it in context. I have had parents tell me they've cut out entire food groups from their child's diet because of one article they read featuring one study. (Dairy comes to mind, which means eliminating calcium, a major source of much-needed minerals for growing kids.)

Fear-based headlines can trigger lots of emotion, particularly when they implicate something we care about as much as our children's health. Yet the details of those emotion-driven headlines and study findings aren't always what they seem. Many studies on diet, for example, show *associations* between eating habits and health outcomes, *not direct cause*. So while we may make what we feel is a health-protecting leap by cutting something out of our diet, we aren't accounting for a whole host of *other* common factors that could cause the outcome. I'm thinking of a study that came in through my email newswire just the other day that boasted "ultra-processed foods cause heart disease" and that each extra weekly serving increased risk by 10 percent. That's enough to make any parent feel guilty for feeding their child chicken nuggets for dinner, allowing them to breakfast on a bowl of cereal, snack on a Z-bar, or enjoy a scoop of ice cream after practice. What parents might not be aware of is the fact that the group studied could have other factors in common that put them at risk for cardiovascular disease—factors that have nothing to do with what they eat. Perhaps those who eat processed foods more often also work more jobs and can't cook from scratch, have more stress, or live alone, which are also all factors that have been linked with heart disease, for example.

Most of the studies we hear about in the news are often taken out of context or are misunderstood and often don't warrant making sweeping changes to the diet. That's particularly so if it means cutting out or eliminating a certain food or food group, since all foods can be an opportunity for nourishment, which is particularly important to a growing child. For most of us, focusing on ensuring our daughters get enough nourishment (i.e., overall calories, vitamins, and minerals) to support growth while also maintaining a positive relationship with food is enough to juggle. It's best to avoid adding on fear-based responsibilities that require close monitoring and instead, focus on the most important task at hand in a positive way.

Of course, you will feel inclined to intervene on their eating with rules or limits every now and again—or maybe even daily. If you're wondering if you're crossing a line, ask yourself if the limit or rules you want to impose might, despite being good for their physical health, harm other aspects of their health. And, if so, is it worth it? For example, telling your daughter that she's had enough cookies at a party might mean she eats less sugar, but it might also cause her some shame, deny her a pleasure that others are freely enjoying, and/or put a dent in her burgeoning eating competence and internal regulation skills. Is that harm worth the benefit of eating a few less grams of sugar? And, yes, you will be right when you explain to your teen that bringing food from home is a more nutritious option than grabbing lunch from the cafeteria with friends. However, if it limits her ability to be feel connected with her peers and results in a lot of residual stress, is that restriction truly keeping her emotionally healthy?

Additionally, when concerns about how their eating might impact their physical health, remind yourself that eating habits are not forever. Remember that children, adolescents, and teens go through developmental stages with regard to their eating, just as they do with other areas of their life. Frustrating as it is, rolling along with their sudden and nonsensical food refusals during the time when they are asserting their independence, giving them the freedom to explore the convenience of packaged foods they see their friends eating during adolescence, and allowing them to try vegetarianism during the experimental teens years can do more to build their eating competence and overall nutritional health over the long term than warning them about the dangers of not eating enough leafy greens or the amount of sodium in a bag of Cheetos. Just like her love of pom-pom headbands doesn't mean she'll be a fashion disaster when she one day decides to work in a hospital or walk into a boardroom, her decision to enjoy a snack of Sour Pour Rainbow Straws does not mean she's destined to be riddled with arthritis, cavities, cardiovascular disease, or diabetes for the rest of her life.

IFM Touchstone: *Well-being*

Which aspect of your daughter's well-being do you prioritize the most? Which one have you overlooked or de-emphasized? What is one small action you can take to help your daughter have a more well-rounded approach to healthy eating? For example, *I intend to remind myself that enjoyment is part of healthy eating;* or *I intend to keep the conversation at the table fun and lighthearted to help make meals together more enjoyable.*

As I got to know Sarah, her family, and her history, I did investigate her changes in BMI percentile. Asking her and mom gentle questions about how life had changed during the time when her body weight started to increase faster than her height shined a light on a fact that I already suspected. In spring of the year prior, Sarah, like my own daughters and millions of others, had a sudden shift in her day-to-day activities, as well as her level of stress. Coinciding with the pandemic, Sarah's physical activity decreased significantly, due at least in part to the fact that she lived in the center of a large urban city with little access to outdoor space. Not surprisingly, her emotional stress abruptly increased as well. She was suddenly isolated from friends and her daily routine, her parents were irritable and unsure, and the highlight of her weekdays—an hour and a half spent ice skating or swimming—ended completely. While her social and emotional stresses increased, her main coping mechanisms—friends and sports—were simultaneously removed completely. Like many people, she was eating more and moving less while experiencing a great amount of emotional turmoil and stress, two factors that situationally and biologically speaking had the potential to prime her body to increase fat stores.

A year and a half later, her emotional and social life was getting back on track—she was back at school and seeing friends, returned to sports, and felt happier and more relaxed. Her BMI had stabilized, a positive sign that in time it would return to its original percentile. She felt happy and relaxed about her eating. If she'd taken on a diet or continued to make it a goal to bring down her weight, I think she'd be in a much different place emotionally, socially, and physically.

REFLECTIONS ON WELL-BEING

- *In the past, which part of your well-being has been the most important to you—physical health, emotional health, or relationships?*

- *Do you think you've emphasized one aspect of your daughter's well-being over others?*

- *If you believe one area is being emphasized over others, do you think bringing more balance to her life could help her have a happier, healthier relationship with food? Do you think it might improve her relationship with her body? If yes, how?*

- *Do you feel like you are more focused on one area of your own well-being? If so, which one and why?*

- *Which area of your well-being are you least focused on? What might the benefit be of focusing on it more? What is one step you can take to do that?*

CHAPTER FIVE
WEIGHT

"Labeling your child as overweight and taking
steps to remedy it, whether direct or indirect, make
her feel flawed and inferior in all ways."

—*Ellyn Satter, Your Child's Weight: Helping Without Harming*

AT LEAST THREE EXTREMELY PERSISTENT AND EQUALLY DAM-
aging beliefs about weight threaten our well-being, particularly if
we are living in or raising daughters living in larger bodies or bodies
defined as "overweight" or "obese" by the body mass index (BMI).
While the topic of weight is not a touchstone of the IFM, it dominates
so much of our unconscious beliefs and attitudes towards eating—even
for those at what's perceived as a normal or "healthy" weight—that I
feel we must dispel these myths if we truly want to protect our daughters from dieting. Let's put misunderstandings about body weight and
BMI to rest once and for all before they begin to haunt our daughters or
continue to haunt us.

First of all, the idea that we have direct control over our weight is
incorrect. Our body weight has a set point where it can rest comfort-
ably, which diets can do little if anything to change—at least over the
long term. We cannot dial our body weight up or down based on our
wishes. Nor can we exert our will over it by changing our eating, at
least not in a way that won't cause significant harm to our physical,
emotional, and mental health. Yes, living in a culture of anti-fat bias

can make this fact difficult to hear or accept. Still, it doesn't help to or ignore it. Instead of allowing your daughter to dwell on this concept as frustrating and unfair, be sure to point out its brilliance. Our body weight is designed to stay in its homeostatic place despite our cruel attempts to starve it. In fact, I'd go as far as to say that the better your daughter's body is at maintaining a stable weight (or BMI percentile in children since, technically, their body weight should be increasing as they grow), the stronger, smarter, and more robust her body will be! In other words, if a body isn't responding well to dieting by diverging from its set point—if it's holding steady despite efforts to shrink it—then it is, in fact, working brilliantly.

Second, the idea that her weight is an indicator of health is incorrect. While we often hear that being overweight is bad for your health, we rarely hear about research that shows just the opposite. For example, a review of 97 studies including more than 2.8 million people published in the prestigious *Journal of the American Medical Association* showed that people in the "obese" BMI category live just as long as those in the "normal" weight category, while those in the "overweight" BMI category lived longer than those living in "normal" weight.[40] Additionally, other studies that do link high BMI with poor health show *associations* only— not *causes*. Further, these studies rarely account for the other issues that negatively impact longevity, such as the stress and stigma people living in larger bodies face when they don't meet idealized cultural standards and the harms of dieting and weight-loss efforts.

Third, the idea that we can fix or change our weight by focusing on food is also incorrect. Weight-loss diets don't just do us wrong by failing us with long-term weight loss; trying to manipulate our weight with food causes nothing but conflict, frustration, and turmoil with our eating, not to mention putting our physical and emotional health at risk. Weight-loss diets, ironically, are also a risk factor for overall weight gain. To be clear, aside from any internalized and externalized anti-fat bias experienced, weight gain or a large body isn't problematic in and of itself; however, for those are considering putting a child through the pain of dieting for the purpose of losing weight it is important to know that the outcome will very likely be the opposite of the one that is being sought. Bottom line: a weight loss diet isn't necessarily a healthy diet and a healthier diet (i.e., one that is more nutritionally sound) isn't necessarily going to cause someone to lose weight.

If you want your daughter to have a healthy relationship with food, enjoy eating habits that are protective and nourishing instead of punitive and malnourishing, and think of her body weight as something positive and immutable, as opposed to something that needs to be corrected or controlled, be vigilant about putting these myths to rest and get support from professionals if and when you or she needs it.

In the rest of this chapter, we'll dive deeper into each of these three myths so that you have a better understanding of how they're harmful. Learning factual information that helps dispel these commons beliefs will also help you communicate a more holistic understanding of weight to your daughter, and stand strong when you come up against others who have yet to do the same.

THE MYTH OF WEIGHT CONTROL

Paramount to building your daughter's confidence, self-acceptance, and self-esteem with her weight is helping her decipher what is in her control and what is not.

To be clear, her body weight is *not* in her direct control. Not in the way she thinks it is. Not in the way the world, her doctors, and dieting experts will tell her it is. In fact, believing that it is and trying to change our weight by focusing on food and extreme exercise or a "calories in, calories out" mentality can have serious and long-lasting repercussions on our health.

Our body weight—and our overall health, for that matter—is determined by an infinitely complex set of factors, including our genetics, metabolic rate, environment, food intake, and activity level. What healthism and diet culture does not tell us is that we have varying levels of control over each of these factors.

When it comes to our genetics, for example, the amount of control we have over them is little to zilch. When it comes to our environment, which includes the literal place we live as well as the economic and social aspects of our surroundings, we have some, but very limited control. Public health experts have significant and long-standing research that proves that a surprisingly vast number of factors in our environment—such as our access and proximity to doctors and dentists, education, jobs, income, food, playgrounds, greens spaces and safe places to be physically active, clean water, and pollution—have more of an impact on our quality of life and longevity than our body weight. In fact, researchers found that the zip code you live in can literally account for as much as a 24 years difference in life expectancy. Yet doctors are much more likely to hand us a prescription for weight loss before ever asking about you or your family's living environment, work schedule, childcare needs, or access to areas to be active.

We do have some degree of control over our food choices and eating behaviors. However, even those are significantly more complicated than weight loss culture would have them seem. You don't just decide to eat less or more or forgo one option for another without repercussions on your hunger, appetite, metabolism, self-esteem, sense of self-worth, happiness, future resources, and more.

Your daughter needs to understand that, even if she skips a few meals and goes low-to-no-carb for a few weeks, she may see the scale move; however, eventually her body will start operating on less energy, meeting her near those lower intake goals. Inevitably, weight loss will slow or stop. Or, her ability to exercise such restraint will catch up to her and eventually she'll be so stressed or hungry or both that she will give in to hunger and feed her body the high-calorie food it has been asking for. Either way, without understanding that her weight isn't exactly in her control, she's likely to regard her body's inability to bend to her will as a personal failure. Or worse, she'll ramp up her efforts to cut back or increase activity even more.

WEIGHT IS NOT A MARKER OF OUR DAUGHTER'S HEALTH

While it flies in the face of everything diet and wellness cultures are telling us, and even contradicts what we hear from the majority of the medical community, a person's body weight is not a direct indicator of their health. Girls in thinner bodies are not necessarily going to live longer than girls in larger bodies, nor are they healthier or extra protected against physical disease. (In fact, at least one study indicated that the thinnest children are at increased risk for health concerns as adults[2].) And girls in larger bodies aren't necessarily unhealthy nor at increased risk for disease.

Yes, there is research that shows that children at higher BMI percentiles and higher abdominal fatness have higher risks of disease and disease risk factors. However, those studies are most often showing associations, not direct causation. Additionally, not all associations are negative, though we rarely hear that side of the story. For one, higher BMI children are shown to have the same risk of disease in adulthood as "normal" weight children. Another reassuring finding seen in some studies: women who carried extra body fat from childhood into adulthood actually were found to have lower triglycerides and cholesterol, two significant factors that confer extra protection against heart disease.[3] And since we are talking BMI, many parents I've worked with get extremely upset and concerned when they see that their child's has risen above a certain cutoff point. Many times, this sudden upset is not necessary. Actually, these cutoff points have been criticized by researchers as being arbitrary numbers with no meaning. According to a study in the *British Medical Journal*, "the 85th or 95th percentile is intrinsically no more valid than the 90th, 91st, 97th, or 98th percentile."[4] In other words, hitting (or sitting at) a certain number on the BMI percentile chart is not necessarily the risk factor for disease that many of us believe it to be. And that is yet another reason we need to look at the whole picture of our child's habits and well-being when it comes to assessing their health as opposed to focusing on their weight.

Another BMI-related matter that can reassure us about our daughter's health is the fact that multiple studies have indicated that people living at BMIs classified as "overweight" *outlive* people living at BMIs classified as "normal."[5]

Of course, none of this information warrants skipping regular medical visits with your child's provider nor any recommended lab tests to detect disease or metabolic dysfunction. Nor is it meant to imply that peer-reviewed, clinical research showing direct causation between weight loss and improved metabolic health are false. This information is meant to reassure you that your daughter's weight or BMI alone is not necessarily an indicator of, nor should it be blamed for, her current or future health. And we should not forcibly reduce it with a harmful practice such as dieting to cure health conditions.

> **Bookmark** *Health at Every Size: The Surprising Truth About Your Weight* by Lindo Bacon, PhD. When people ask me for evidence that weight loss is not an effective strategy for increasing overall health or specific conditions, I recommend they check out Chapter 6: "We're Victims of Fat Politics," or an academic paper that appeared in 2011 in the *Nutrition Journal* called "Weight Science: Evaluating the Evidence for a Paradigm Shift" also by Bacon and fellow weight science researcher Lucy Aphramor, RD, which a simple google search can help you find.[6]

DIETING DOES THE DAMAGE

When we dig deeper into the research on weight management interventions and when we listen closely to the stories of people who've been trying to push down the number on the scale for decades, we can see clearly that the business of trying to shrink the body is often futile—and even harmful. When we come to understand the very low possibility of weight loss attempts succeeding over the long term and acknowledge the harm of trying to reduce our child's body size, the fact that health-care experts recommend it at all, frankly, makes no sense.

Pediatricians, in particular, are advised to avoid making overt recommendations for weight loss for their patients since research indicates that there are significant risks in dieting, particularly for children. In fact, as I mentioned in the previous chapter, pediatricians have been advised to avoid talking about or focusing on weight at all. Yet, based on the stories I hear from parents and teens, many of them still do.

"In our eating disorders clinic, we see children who were told by their doctor that they need to lose weight and then they may even bring their BMI down to the 50th percentile, which is considered 'healthy' but they are very, very sick," explains Tracy Richmond, MD, MPH, director of the Eating Disorder Program at Boston Children's Hospital.

When we try to force down our weight, we do damage to our emotional and physical welfare as well as our long-term relationship with food. Interestingly, adolescents at higher BMIs are more likely to suffer from eating disorders, probably due to the fact that they're more likely to try a diet.[7] Dieting is a significant risk factor for eating disorders. In one large three-year-long study, adolescent girls ages 14 to 15 who tried to diet (i.e., restricted calories or skipped meals) were 18 times more likely to go on to develop an eating disorder.[8] Girls in the same study who dieted but not as strictly or severely were five times more likely to develop an eating disorder. Even if dieting did prove successful at helping a person lose and keep off unwanted weight (which it doesn't), and even if losing weight cured kids of diseases (which it can't necessarily do), the astounding risk of developing a secondary condition as life-threatening as an eating disorder is reason enough to go to great lengths to protect your daughter from trying one herself.

Of course, your daughter doesn't need to suffer from a full-blown eating disorder to get hurt by dieting. Weight loss diets aren't just internally torturous and uncomfortable; they cause harm in multiple other ways, too. If you're raising a daughter who is living in a body that doesn't conform to cultural ideals or is at a higher BMI, then your resolve to avoid a weight loss diet will be tested time and time again. Thus, I've compiled a longer list of facts to help you feel reassured that it's best to avoid that urge. You can use these reasons to protect yourself against societal pressure, as well as share them with your daughter if and when she insists on embarking on a weight loss diet herself.

UNDERSTANDING WHAT'S BEST TO FOCUS ON

While we may not have direct control over our body weight, your daughter will also do well to understand those things she does have at least some, if not all, control over. These include her day-to-day habits, which can enhance her health regardless of independent weight loss.

For example, we can choose to focus on making movement (if it is available to us) a priority—and choose how we like to move to increase the likelihood we will stick to it. We can set aside time to destress. We can seek out relationships that are positive, supportive, and affirming, and avoid those that aren't. We can choose to prioritize sleep over other distractions like watching Netflix and scrolling through social media. We can focus on positive eating habits, such as eating meals prepared at home if and when possible, planning meals ahead of time, eating intuitively, and making an effort to eat together with our children if that time is available to us (based on our schedules), as opposed to demonizing, restricting, limiting foods, or skipping meals.

All of the above habits, by the way, are linked with many of the same health benefits that weight loss is usually miscredited for, including lowered risk of heart disease and diabetes, reduced inflammation, better blood sugar control, increased nutrient intake, improved mood and memory, and a longer life.

Once I convince a parent that a weight loss diet isn't the best approach for their child when it comes to improving health and wellbeing, these are the health-promoting habits I recommend they reorient their daughters' attention towards. Prioritizing and developing these habits will lead to much greater and longer-term health benefits than a weight loss diet. The following specific areas can work to directly improve or protect our daughters' health *regardless of their impact on her body weight*.

Regular, Enjoyable Physical Activity has been shown to increase muscle cells' sensitivity to insulin, making them more efficient at using glucose (a.k.a. carbohydrates) for energy, which means better blood sugar control and lower risk of insulin resistance for those who are prone to it; help regulate hunger and fullness hormones, improving our ability to be attuned to how much or how little we need to eat to meet our day-to-day energy needs; reduce inflammation, which has been identified as a root cause of multiple diseases and dysfunction, including heart disease and cancer; improve blood flow, lowering the risk of heart disease; lower blood pressure; lower triglycerides and total cholesterol by reducing low-density lipoprotein (LDL- or bad cholesterol) and increasing high-density lipoprotein (HDL, or good cholesterol); increase bone density; reduce oxidative stress that would otherwise cause brain cell function decline and is likely why exercise is associated with better memory and cognition in kids; up brain sensitivity to feel-good chemicals such as dopamine, increasing the ability to feel joy; and, increase growth in a specific part of the brain that protects against (and reverses) mood disorders such as depression.[9] Note that these benefits are seen at low-to-moderate levels of regular exercise; physical activity that is high in frequency, duration, or intensity may not have similar benefits. If your child has limited physical ability to be active, I recommend seeking out trusted support in how to do modified or ability-appropriate activity either online or in-person as opposed to avoiding it altogether.

Sufficient Sleep: Sleep deprivation (or a lack of regular, deep sleep) reduces the body's ability to regulate blood sugar, lowers immune function, increases the drive for caloric energy, dysregulates hormones, and decreases brain function, making us more susceptible to low moods and depression.[10] Consequently, focusing on making sure our kids are getting enough sleep and quality sleep can protect against all those things.

Positive Relationships: Not feeling connected to others has been shown to decrease immune function, raise blood pressure, and increase cortisol, a stress hormone—three factors that increase the risk of disease such as diabetes. Helping your daughter cultivate positive relationships can reduce the risk of those disease-causing factors.

Stress Management: Chronic stress has been shown to decrease immune function; increase blood pressure and inflammation; and alter hormones and normal digestion in multiple ways, including appetite.[11] All these changes can ramp up disease risk individually and collectively, which is why supporting our daughters in recognizing and reducing psychological distress is protective against these diseases.

Fruits, Vegetables, Grains, and Plant-Based Fats: These food groups in particular contain antioxidants, vitamins, minerals, fiber, and polyunsaturated and monounsaturated fats that reduce blood pressure, inflammation, and oxidative stress, as well as help balance blood sugar. All of these changes are linked with lower risk of multiple diseases, which is why eating these foods is protective. (More on when and how to start focusing on these foods in Chapter 8 on Nutrition.)

GETTING POSITIVE HEALTHCARE & SUPPORT

If your daughter is living in a larger body, has a BMI percentile that has been steadily rising, or has recently seemed to have gained more weight than you think is "normal" for her age, you might be feeling anxious about her next medical visit. If she has already been diagnosed with a disease or condition, such as type 2 diabetes, prediabetes, insulin resistance, or polycystic ovary syndrome (PCOS), you may be concerned that the medical experts you need to confer with to help you manage the condition will make her feel bad or shamed about her weight. You may worry that they will continue to push for weight loss despite evidence that this approach can be harmful. Unfortunately, that's a legitimate concern, since the majority of providers are trained to see high BMI and high BMI percentiles as a problem.

Despite the challenge in getting medical care that takes into account your child's overall well-being, I never suggest ignoring or minimizing these conditions. What I suggest is that you find a provider who believes—like I do—that your child's health will be best served if we avoid "treating" their body weight as if it, in and of itself, is causing the problem and instead, focus on and treat the condition or conditions she has been diagnosed with, preferably with an emphasis on changing or improving habits such as those mentioned in the previous section.

Finding a provider who will recommend health interventions that don't focus on or make her feel bad about her body shape or size will be a key in helping her get the support that will benefit her physical health and overall well-being. One way to do this is by looking for providers who refer to themselves as having a weight-inclusive or Health at Every Size® (HAES®)-aligned or informed approach to health care. (For more information about HAES®, visit the Association for Size Diversity and Health at www.asdah.org.) Typically, unlike many mainstream providers, these professionals won't make the mistake of trying to treat her condition by focusing on a diet or telling her she will be happier and healthier if she loses weight. Nutritionists, dietitians, endocrinologists, and psychotherapists are just a few of the types of providers who identify as HAES®-aligned.

If your daughter has been given a clean bill of health from a provider and weight gain is your only concern, continue to remind yourself that a diet is never the answer. Be mindful of the urge to make changes to her eating under the guise of helping her be "healthier." If the goal is weight loss, then any interference with her eating can be considered dieting and will ultimately be a harmful impact on her health and self-esteem. (I'm reiterating this point because if your daughter is visibly gaining weight beyond what is expected there's a good chance that pressure from the outside world will continually insist that you address it. Maintain your resolve to protect her from this harm. You can rely on your IFM to help you do it.)

If you believe her weight increases are beyond what would be normal for her age and developmental stage, I recommend enlisting the help of a registered dietitian trained by the Satter Institute (visit ellynsatterinstitute.org or email amelia@ameliasherry.com and I can help you connect with someone in your area.) A professional can carefully assess and identify any possible medical, developmental, nutritional, psychosocial, and family feeding dynamics that might be contributing to the change in your daughter's expected weight gain trajectory and correct them. They can also refer you to other sources of support (such as therapists, parent groups, and medical specialists if needed).

QUESTIONS TO ASK PROVIDERS

While I wish that all providers were weight inclusive, at the time of writing this book, that is not the case. Understanding how a practitioner views weight in the context of overall health *before* you are seen by them is important. "Questions such as the following can go a long way in making sure that you're not setting up an appointment with someone who is going to reinforce weight stigma for you or your daughter," says Brianna Clark, LCSW, a New York based psychotherapist and eating-disorder expert:

5. Is the doctor I will be seeing a HAES®-aligned clinician? If not, are they HAES®-informed and willing to take that approach with patients who request it? (If they are, ask to explicitly make that request now and have it noted for your initial appointment.)

6. How does your practice navigate patient requests to not be weighed at their appointments? (In the case of annual well visits for children when information is added to the growth chart, are blind weights available?)

7. What are my options if I do not feel comfortable with the provider I see at my initial appointment?

8. What steps does this practice take to ensure non-weight-stigmatizing care for all its patients?

• •

Another point Clark recommends keeping in mind is the need to be willing to expand your search area beyond the usual geographic limits. "One of the silver linings of the Covid-19 pandemic is an increased prevalence of telehealth options for diagnosis and symptom management, and overall health maintenance (depending, of course, on the specifics of your healthcare needs). If your health concerns align with your provider's telehealth treatment guidelines, you may be able to minimize your in-person trips to a faraway provider and utilize telehealth for maintenance appointments instead," explains Clark. And she adds that there's an added bonus of telehealth appointments—no routine weigh-ins!

GROWTH CHARTS: WHAT AM I LOOKING AT?

At some point during my career as an endocrine dietitian, I attended a lecture on growth. During one of the presentations, someone stood on the stage, pointed to a growth chart and said, "Healthy children grow in predictable ways." It was an aha moment for me; I found the statement as clarifying as it was reassuring, and I share it with the parents I work with often. This fact is reiterated and explained in several of Satter's books. I have come to rely on it as one way to help reassure parents that they don't need to "fix" their child's weight. You might wonder, *what does it mean?*

Many children who are developmentally healthy—meaning without a significant diagnosis of disease or genetic syndrome—grow in a very predictable pattern. This pattern is seen reflected in all forms of the basic growth chart (e.g., height, weight, BMI, and for younger children, head circumference). While I don't agree with the idea that our BMI

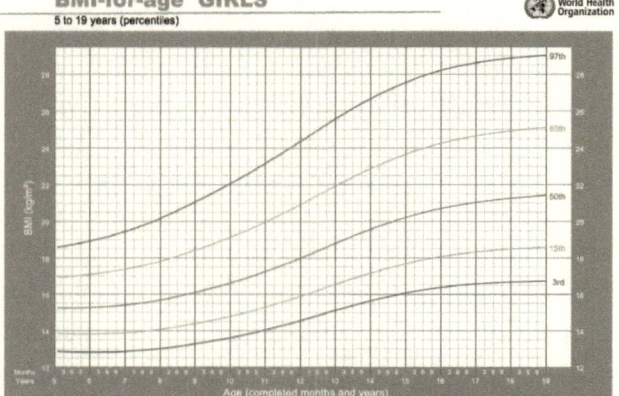

BMI-for-age GIRLS
5 to 19 years (percentiles)

Figure 5.1

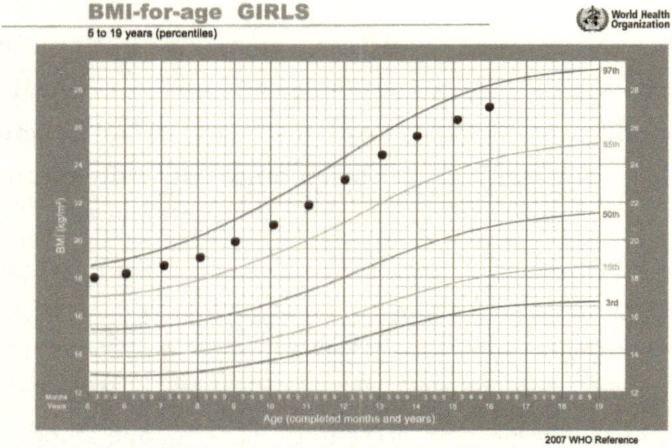

BMI-for-age GIRLS
5 to 19 years (percentiles)

Figure 5.2

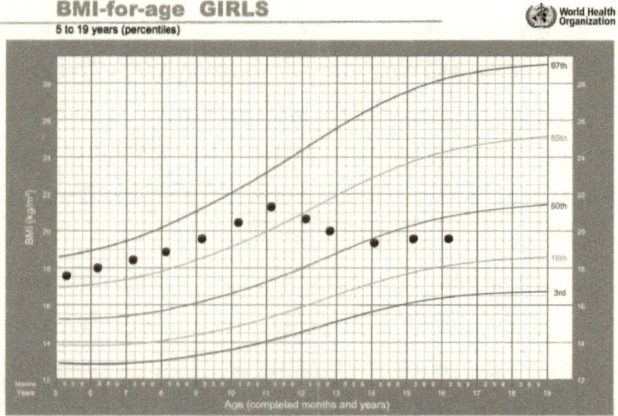

BMI-for-age GIRLS
5 to 19 years (percentiles)

Figure 5.3

defines our health, the BMI percentile charts for children have proved to be of value to me in helping to evaluate a child's growth and health.

If you look at a standard BMI chart (see Figure 5.1), you can see that as a child ages, their BMI tends to increase, following a steady "curve" throughout her life. Where the line is flatter (from ages five to six, for example), it typically increases more slowly. Where the line is steeper (from ages 11 to 12 years), it typically will increase more rapidly. That is to say that during those years, a girl is expected to grow more rapidly in weight than in height.

For many parents, when we're told that our child's BMI, or height or weight or head circumference is at a high percentile, we have feelings about it. Like, *strong* feelings. We worry, or we're proud, or we're reassured. Or we freak out and start googling furiously, which is exactly what I did after being told the circumference of my eldest daughter's head was extremely high and something we needed to "watch." (As it turns out, my husband's family just have big heads—and my daughter has that genetic destiny, too. Her head was larger than average, but followed its curve, growing just as predicted.)

Similarly, some kids are just in larger bodies. What I explain to anxious parents raising kids above the 85th and below the 20th percentile is that so long as your child is "hugging their curve," they are doing just fine.

In other words, if your daughter is at the 90th percentile for BMI and has been holding steady there since she was five, that's not a problem. It's normal and healthy, in fact. She's growing predictably and, remember, "healthy children grow in predictable ways." (See Figure 5.2) She does not need to eat less or workout more or worry that her BMI alone will put her at risk for diabetes, cancer, and heart disease.

On the other hand, if she was plotting there and we suddenly saw a dip down to the 50th percentile (see Figure 5.3), or what would be considered a more average and "normal" number, it would be a cause for serious alarm. Something significant in her eating, activity, environment, or habits would have had a change, and she likely would be at risk for those malnutrition risks discussed earlier in the chapter.

The same goes for girls in smaller bodies. I've seen girls (and boys) at below the 5th percentile who are referred to me for malnutrition, and yet, regardless of their below-average intake of overall calories, they are following the curve in a predictable way and thriving in other areas of development. These kids have been above-average students and musicians, they are outgoing, and in some cases, can analyze more plot lines in *Harry Potter* than Emma Watson herself. Yes, they are living in a body that is outside of the "normal" BMI, yet there's no reason to believe there's anything unhealthy about them. Again, some kids are genetically designed to live in smaller or leaner bodies. As Satter says so bluntly, "Some children are short and stocky, some children are tall and slender. Some children are fat, and some are thin. Your child's size and shape are determined mostly by heredity: the size and shape of her mother and father. Expect her to grow according to her genes, not to your wishes."[12] (Pronouns changed)

While we can assume that as long as a child is staying steady on their curve, they are doing pretty well with their eating; what we do need to take note of are detours from that curve. With regard to BMI in particular, falling off that line or suddenly veering up is a change we need to investigate. This is an important and sometimes confusing point to note, so listen closely here: If your child has been hugging her curve at a high BMI—above the "normal" range—and suddenly takes a dive down into the "normal" range, that is not normal for your child and needs to be looked at further.

While a change upwards is more likely to be noted and worried about by a healthcare provider, *any* significant deviation from the curve should be investigated further by a health professional such as a pediatrician or pediatric endocrinologist, as well as a pediatric dietitian. It's not always an indicator of a problem, but it is worth looking into. In many cases, holding a line, no matter what the percentile (less than the 5th to above the 90th), can be an indication that the child is growing normally and is healthy. Veering off—whether upwards or downwards or into or out of a "normal" range—on any of the charts (height, weight,

BMI) deserves additional attention. Remember, *healthy children grow in predictable ways.*

We want to dig until we can figure out the *cause* of the change, not focus on a diet to erase the result of the change. We want to address that change in a positive way that leaves the goal of reversing her weight out of the equation. Just remember, even if your daughter has veered up off that curve, a weight loss diet is still not the healthy or healthiest solution.

REFLECTIONS ON WEIGHT

- *When it comes to your daughter's weight, what is your biggest concern?*

- *How is focusing on her weight helping her? (Is it helping her with her relationship with food? With her self-esteem? With her relationship with her body? With her habits? With her health?)*

- *How might focusing on her weight be harming her?*

- *If you have a copy of your daughter's BMI chart, can you tell if her BMI percentile has stayed relatively steady? If it has changed, can you see roughly the time when it started to do so? If yes, do you remember any changes that happened around that time (environment such as a move or school, social such as friends or family, or physical such as the start of a new medication)?*

- *If you were to put weight to the side, are there any habits that you think your daughter could benefit from doing more or less of? In what ways (unrelated to weight) might that change (or changes) benefit her?*

CHAPTER SIX
TRUST

"Our inner guidance comes to us through our feelings and body
wisdom first—not through intellectual understanding."

—*Christine Northrup*

MANY YEARS AGO, MY OLDER BROTHER AND I WERE ON A RARE
bike ride together, exploring the sandy roads of Martha's
Vineyard. At some point, we stopped to get some lunch. We walked
towards an aluminum bike rack and pushed our front tires through the
rails to rest. I watched as he pulled a flimsy metal cord with a little
luggage lock out of his backpack. He wound it around the neck of our
bikes, through the spokes, and then attached it to the rack.

I was irritated.

The thought of having to lock up our things in this beautiful,
relaxed, and sacred-feeling place felt wrong. "What's that little thing
going to do anyway?" I snipped.

"This just keeps an honest person honest," he answered surely, with
a bit of chuckle. Irritating his little sister was a game, which heightened
my indignation toward the lock even more.

All through lunch, I stared at the shiny cord wrapped around the
stem of my bike like a noose. I ran my eyes over the other bikes, leaning
free. I watched the fishermen in their tall rubber boots working the
boats at the dock, the two children drawing in the sand with sticks, the

weathered boards of the building we sat outside of, and my toes digging down and up through the sand. I ignored most of what he was saying and listened to the ocean waves rising and falling instead. I remember thinking about how the waves had nothing to worry about but the moon. I watched some teenagers walk into the sandwich shop without any shoes on.

"You know, the only thing that thing does is scream, 'We don't trust you!'" I snarled, having spent the entire time it took him to eat a turkey sandwich to build my case. "'The best way to find out if you can trust somebody is to *trust them.*' Haven't you ever heard that before?"

My brother looked confused, probably wondering why I was quoting Hemingway instead of what in heaven I was riled up about.

"The lock!" I reminded him. "It says more about you than anything else. You're telling people you don't trust them."

He smirked and rolled his eyes. And I'm guessing he never gave it another thought that day or any day since. The lesson stayed with me, though.

Every time I see my husband put chocolate up on the tippy top shelf of our cupboard, or I find myself stowing a jar of Nutella in the waaaay, way back of the fridge, behind the tomato sauce and long-forgotten jar of pickles that no one ever eats, I think about that bike lock.

Is hiding tempting food out of sight a strategy that'll keep us all honest about what we eat? Or am I simply telling my kids, who always seem to know exactly what my husband and I are doing, "I can't trust you with this." If I truly want my daughters to feel self-trust—and trusted—around certain foods, then I must stop sending them subtle signals that they're aren't trustworthy.

THE NOT-SO-OBVIOUS FACT ABOUT EATING

While it's too rarely talked about or taught, trust is one of the most vital parts of being and raising a healthy eater. And that, my friend, is something I think all us parents need to understand above everything else. Before we learned about never giving an infant honey, that they're ready for solids when they start reaching or grabbing for your food, or that grapes and hot dogs need to be cut in tiny pieces, we would have done well to know that in many cases trusting our child—and supporting them in trusting themselves—is key when it comes to healthy feeding.

A second piece of info I think us parents would have benefitted from knowing: Eating can be broken into two distinct parts. There are the parts of eating we *learn* and parts that we *know* in our bodies. If we as parents understand which eating skills are learned and which are intuitive, instinctual, and body-led, then we can more easily know how best to approach many tough decisions about feeding, including when to allow sweets and treats and whether or how much we should insist they eat foods like fruits and vegetables. (For children born with significant health issues, developmental delays, or neurodiversity, these two parts of eating may be interrupted, take work to restore, or require adaptive efforts. Regardless of challenges, I think parents benefit from understanding this as a basic concept eating just as much as the expectation that an infant will one day progress from liquids and purees to solids.) When it comes to those aspects of eating that we all do cognitively and thus, need to learn and grow with in time, we need to lean in with support and leadership. And when it comes to those things we can only know with our bodies, we parents need to lean out and relax, giving our kids an opportunity to turn inward and figure things out using their own body's natural instincts. Leading with trust is key to helping our kids master both of these areas of eating.

The problem is that many social and cultural pressures interfere with how we understand, approach, and think about eating and feeding our children. As you will learn in this chapter, many health edicts and recommendations for feeding kids (and ourselves!) tell us to lean in and out at all the wrong times and in the wrong ways.

When it comes to eating and feeding, here are examples of the times it's best to let go of control and where our kids benefit most if we tighten the reins. I will also share some insights into the sneaky things that tend to undermine our ability to do this, and finally, a tool that can make figuring it all out a whole lot easier!

EATING SKILLS WE KNOW

Your daughter was born with a certain kind of eating genius. And so were you! That is to say that your daughter—like all healthy infants— was born with a natural ability to regulate her daily energy intake. This *knowing* encompasses the body-led, or somatic, skills of eating and is information that the body does best to *sense* or *feel*, as opposed to *think*, its way through. That means that from the moment we are born, the vast majority of us have the innate skill of knowing exactly how few or many calories we need to consume on any given day in response to our activity and growth needs.[1]

If you've ever read up on the reciprocal biochemistry of breastfeeding, you're probably already aware of the responsiveness or *knowing* that a mother's body shows towards her infant. A nursing mother's breast milk changes in protein, fat, and carbohydrate content as her growing infant's nutritional needs change. Research shows that the composition of breastmilk even changes on an hourly basis in tune with circadian rhythms, producing a more energy-rich mix in the morning and a more soothing one at night.[2] If one body can respond to another body's needs in this way, imagine the *knowing* ability it can show towards itself.

Our bodies are responsive to the energy *density* of foods (for example, if a food is particularly high in fat and calories) throughout life and, if we are listening with our body or sensing it, adjust our intake based on those measures. Most of us can identify with the feeling, for example, of eating a particularly high fat, high calorie, energy dense, or "heavy" meal at lunch and feeling less hungry at dinner. Or noticing that after a long day spent playing outside, swimming, or running around with friends, our daughter's appetite seems to surge. Our energy needs ebb and flow from age to age and from growth spurt to times of slower growth, as well as from day to day throughout life, based on a multitude of factors including activity, stress level, sickness, social factors, type and timing of foods eaten at the previous meal, and our own history with food. When we are attuned to our body or listening closely, we can feel our appetite change in tune with our day-to-day calorie needs.

Thank heaven our body has this miraculous ability to *know* or sense how much we need; otherwise, could you imagine from meal to meal, day after day having to stop and calculate the exact right number of calories to eat based on a multitude of factors such as your age, exact time in your menstrual cycle, the number of steps taken or stairs climbed, nutrients, and quantities eaten earlier?

The fact that our body knows how much or how little to eat is an important one, not only to understand and embrace, but also to share with our tween and teen daughters, who might otherwise be convinced that they need to eat small portions or on a very specific schedule according a TikTok star's recommendations, a book-based plan, or a comparison between herself and her friends. No one can ever explain to her how to feel full and satisfied with a specific number of grapes, gulps of milk, or forkfuls of pasta, just as they couldn't tell her how to like the creamy texture of a perfectly ripened avocado or the tart sweetness of a raspberry or the salty crunch of a tortilla chip. Her body senses this kind of information based on a host of ever-changing factors at a speed that our brains could never outpace. What one person needs to eat to feel full and satisfied in one day does not translate to what is true for another. (You will learn more about nutritional needs to keep our daughters well-nourished in Chapter 8.)

The somatic skills of eating are the things we *sense* or *feel*, as opposed to *think*, our way through. The *knowing* of parts of eating—the parts we do best when we listen to our bodies—includes deciding how much or how little to eat of any given food at any given meal, as well as whether we like it or not. Luckily, the majority of healthy kids *know* how to handle the how much and how little of eating like champs from the moment they are born. Our only job here as parents and feeders is not to teach them how to eat the exact right portion—it is to consistently and authentically *trust* that they can do it.

. . . .

SPECIAL SITUATIONS

While the majority of healthy children (and adults) can use their body sensations to *know* how much or how little to eat, for a smaller group of people that might not be possible. For those with eating disorders (or disordered eating including chronic dieting), taking medications that interrupt or exaggerate hunger and fullness signals, or who have diagnoses such as Autism Spectrum Disorder (ASD), Attention Deficit Hyperactivity Disorder (ADHD), or a genetic syndrome such as Prader-Willi, connecting to body sensations that help us regulate our food intake can be more difficult. If your daughter falls into one or more of these categories, talk to a registered dietitian or feeding specialist who can explain more about how and why these connections are disrupted, as well as offer you other positive ways to help her manage eating just the right amounts.

. . . .

CULTIVATING OUR OWN EATING KNOWING

When I first learned the fact that a child can regulate their own food intake with precision and accuracy, I was still deep in the suffering of my dieting days. The idea that at one point in my life I may have had a certain body knowing or genius about eating was both as mind-boggling and inconceivable as it was profound and therapeutic. *You mean I was once good at eating? Perhaps my dieting—not genetics or lack of willpower—is what stole that from me? Ridiculous! How could these heavy thighs be healthy?* I wrestled with it at first; it seemed implausible. And in my disordered mind of the time, I was definitely not going to risk weight gain to find out.

Yet as the years went on and my understanding of the things that may have contributed to my distrust of my hunger also helped me regain my body esteem, the idea of this inner knowing reeked suspiciously of, well, common sense. *My body knows? Or used to know, at least? Of course it did! What else could explain the fact that people ate perfectly well within their needs (when food was available, at least) during those billions of years before measuring cups and calorie counting apps existed?*

By the time I discovered the book on the concept of intuitive eating around 2006 or 2007, I was ready to listen. I had more respect for my body and reverence for what it was capable of, and with that in mind, I wanted nothing but to recapture my inborn ability to *know*. Discovering the concept of intuitive eating as explained by dietitians Evelyn Tribole and Elyse Resch was a major turning point for me; it gave me the framework, guidance, and tactical skills I needed to do it—plus the research I needed to believe in it when it felt scary, hard, or wrong.

To date, there have been about 200 individual studies on intuitive eating. According to one review analyzing the results of 26 of these studies, researchers concluded that use of intuitive eating was inversely associated with BMI, helped users maintain their weight (though not necessarily lose it), improved mental health, lowered blood pressure and cholesterol levels, and improved their nutrient intake and eating behaviors. All the studies included in the review defined intuitive eating as eating when hungry, stopping eating when no longer hungry or when full, and having no restrictions on the types of foods eaten (except in cases of medical conditions). People who approach eating this way experience benefits in other areas of their eating too, including being more accepting of new foods, having more relaxed attitudes and open minds about foods (thus, they are exposed to a greater variety of foods and more diverse nutrients, as well as being protected from the nutritional deficiencies of eating too few foods). They are also better with planning and preparing meals and more consistent about feeding themselves and their families.

At the core of intuitive eating is the goal of cultivating self-trust with food. To do so, you must allow yourself full permission to enjoy the kinds and amounts you enjoy. For those of us who have been heavily wooed and swayed by the ideas of good foods and bad foods, healthy foods and unhealthy foods, fattening foods and non-fattening foods, this idea of full permission can be liberating, yet also challenging to embrace for ourselves—never mind giving the same permission to our children. Most weight loss and health diets, as well as traditional food parenting practices (such as "clean your plate" or "eat your vegetables before dessert") are deeply predicated on distrust, making the idea that we do best without limits or rules around food difficult to budge from our brains. Still, those limits and fears about foods and fatness are what get us into trouble, as we've already learned.

Giving into the notion of permission with food—as opposed to limits and restrictions—is crucial when it comes to taking back self-trust. The more you can do this for your daughter, the better she'll be able to remain in touch with her own knowing around the right amounts to eat. And if you're struggling to regain this skill yourself, the silver lining is that you've now got extra motivation to be vigilant in not allowing anything to threaten to disconnect her from her own inner knowing in the first place.

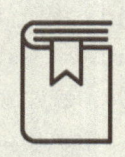 **Bookmark:** To heal your own relationship with food, do a deep dive into *Intuitive Eating: A Revolutionary Anti-Diet Approach* by Evelyn Tribole, MS, RD, CEDRD-S and Elyse Resch, RDN, CEDRD-S, FAND. This book is considered the bible on intuitive eating and helping you understand how to stay tapped into your own eating knowing and heal from the dieting and healthy-eating-at-all-costs mentality for good.

PARENTS PROTECT KNOWING

As mothers who want to protect our daughters from the damages of dieting, our job isn't to figure out how to teach them to be intuitive eaters, but rather to ensure that they *stay* intuitive eaters. And to protect that intuitive knowing, we need to embrace trust by offering full permission.

When we protect our daughter's eating genius, we don't just help her enjoy foods more or avoid an eating disorder. Children who are given permission to eat as much or as little as they like and to grow into the body that is right for them do better with other aspects of eating, too. Ironically, they do better in internal regulation, are better able to accept and enjoy new foods over time, and feel better about their eating overall. Also, thanks to the fact that they feel more confident and positive about their eating, as they get older, they are more likely to feed themselves regularly and reliably, choose balanced meals without much stress or concern, avoid dieting and skipping meals, and enjoy food without guilt or remorse.

As parents we want to do all we can to protect their *knowing* by offering full permission with food. Here's one key: Full permission with food doesn't mean being neglectful or leading with an anything-goes-attitude. Far from it! Our daughters (particularly younger kids) need sufficient guidance and support to stay in touch with *knowing* as they grow from infants to toddlers to school age and beyond. Further in this chapter, you will learn about a tool you can use to help you offer full permission with foods to help her stay in touch with her ability to eat intuitively in a safe and structured way. From my experience, this tool is the best way we as mothers can offer the guidance and support our daughters need to remain in touch with and cultivate knowing as our children grow.

Also, full permission and trusting her knowing doesn't mean we blind ourselves to off-track eating behaviors. If we know that our daughter's BMI percentile is significantly increasing (or decreasing) from where it had been tracking, for example, we can use this as a clue that something significant has changed with her eating. Perhaps she had been internally regulating or using her eating *knowing* quite well for years, then suddenly there's a blip up or a dip down on her growth curve. In this case, our responsibility is to get curious and investigate what may have impacted her ability to stay well-attuned to that knowing. It could be a medical, environmental, or social change, such as a hormonal or digestive issue, a change in school or routine, worries about weight or health, or with stress with a relationship. While many may think the best way to fix this BMI change is to rush in with a special diet, I disagree. Instead, once a medical reason has been ruled out, a smarter parent asks herself if any other factors may be causing a disconnect between her and her eating *knowing*. For example, is it possible that she's been relying on food for emotional relief (see evasive eating in Chapter 4) or started restricting because of pressure from diet culture or worry about her weight? Is she stressed for time and eating on the fly?

The best way to support her in these situations is to help her reconnect with her eating *knowing* as opposed to using outside rules and regulations, such as teaching her to follow portion sizes or insisting she eat more lower (or higher) calorie foods. (Teaching her to rely on outside cues such as those can disconnect her from her body sensations and *eating knowing* even further, worsening the problem.)

EATING SKILLS WE LEARN

While some parts of eating are best guided by our own body trust and *knowing*, there are other aspects of eating that we *learn* from the time we are very young and continually expand on as we age.

For example, we aren't born knowing how to use a spoon and fork, drink with a straw, or sip from a cup. We need to learn those habits via modeling and practice. We also need to *learn* which foods are safe to eat and which are not; again, with guidance and direction from responsible caregivers and feeders. That slice of apple on your plate, for example? Safe. That Lego on the floor? Or goose poop about a foot from the picnic blanket? Not safe. (Although, it turns out, it won't kill your one-year-old if she happens to put it in her mouth during an otherwise lovely summertime picnic when you weren't looking. I won't tell you how I know.) And unless they've been exposed frequently in the womb or through breastmilk, children are not born loving the pungent flavor of garlic, nor spice of curry, nor the bitterness of greens. Appreciating those flavors is something they may or may not learn in time. (A preference for sweet-tasting foods may be prewired in the brain thanks to our innate ability to know sugary foods provide a quick, reliable source of energy, however, so that's at least one thing we can take off our list when it comes to what we need to learn or teach our kids.)

As we grow, we learn about more sophisticated parts of eating and feeding ourselves well. The fact that a mixture of starch, protein, and fat is considered a balanced meal while a bag of Pirate's Booty is not, or that it's important to sit down to eat, or the importance of planning ahead by keeping a stocked pantry or fridge—these are all things we don't come out of the womb knowing, but rather learn as we grow. In fact, many of us (including dietitians) are still learning and perfecting some of the most grown-up skills of eating, such as how to efficiently plan, shop for, and prepare meals for ourselves and others.

Although we may continue learning and perfecting our planning and preparation skills for decades to come, we give our girls the greatest shot at being happy, healthy eaters if we make opportunities for them to learn the importance of prioritizing, planning, and preparing foods for *themselves* to eat when they are young. (Whether or not they want to take on the responsibilities of feeding others—and I pray that they will—is something they can each decide for themselves when they are older.)

The best way to teach some of the more practical or grown-up skills of eating is to lead with a consistent example. Just like you don't need to give your child a doctorate-level education in the safety of certain foods, but rather eat them with and in front of her, you also don't need to get into a big explanation about the benefits of fiber or potential consequences of a diet high in saturated fats or refined sugar. In fact, I have found that children with too much nutrition information can get rather paralyzed by those bits when it comes to making eating decisions, which need to be based on joy and pleasure rather than numbers and facts. For some kids (and adults), taking into account the nutrient composition and potential benefits and harms of food while making decisions about eating can be easy, matter-of-fact, and uncomplicated. For others, it can be wrought with second-guessing, internal conflict, and emotional mayhem, and ultimately lead to eating dysfunction and disorder. Since we don't yet know which of these types of people your daughter is, it's best to keep things positive and simple. From my experience, our daughters have a better shot at being well-nourished, confident, and well-adjusted eaters when parents resist the temptation to overexplain and overcomplicate the nutritional aspects of any given food or eating decision.

PARENTS TRUST THE ABILITY TO LEARN

What would you guess is at the bottom of being good at helping your daughter with all the *learned* skills of eating? It's not being a *Le Cordon Bleu*-trained chef or having the meal-prep skills of someone who's regularly in charge of feeding a small battalion. It's, once again, leaning into trust.

Our job as parents is to give our kids plenty of opportunities to learn in safe and positive environments (a picnic blanket surrounded by geese *not* being one of them) and then trust that they can do it. Just like everything else your child needs to learn, being patient, positive, and trusting is a surefire way for getting great results. Trusting our daughter's ability to learn, even if it is at a slower-than-we'd-like-pace, is key to her actually feeling that she can do it. That means offering a variety of foods regularly and reliably in a pleasant, non-pressured environment so she can push boundaries and explore, and by tasting a new food or helping with cooking, when and if she is ready.

I see so many parents get frustrated with their child's eating skills improving too slowly—they're not eating enough vegetables or learning to like new proteins, or they're not using sauces in the exact right amount—and they share their own disappointment and displeasure with that progress, which undermines their kids' confidence with food and self-esteem about being a "good" eater. One of the questions I ask many of the kids I work with—particularly younger ones when it is not always apparent—is "How do you *feel* about your eating?" Many kids have told me they are "bad" at it and when I've asked why, they cite reasons like "I don't like vegetables" or "I eat too much candy." It's unfortunate, because while the number of vegetables they currently eat is unlikely to have a health impact that will linger for months or years, the way they *feel* about their eating will.

Just like we gave our girls the benefit of doubt when it came to the fact that they would one day learn to crawl, walk, talk, swim, read, write, or learn to ride a bike, it helps if we are positive, patient, and *expectant of eventual success* in the area of eating. When we give our daughters the freedom to make mistakes with food, we are handing them a powerful opportunity to learn what it means to be stuffed or still hungry in their own bodies and for themselves. We also are sending them a silent signal of confidence that we trust they will learn and believe they can do it. We need to stay positive and remind ourselves that they will evolve and hold firm in our belief they have the ability to be happy, healthy eaters even if they aren't there *yet*.

When we trust them to figure it out, they understand that they are trustworthy, capable, confident, and good—feelings that we all want our daughters to have and may extend well beyond their eating. We also give them valuable opportunities to make their own missteps. For example, giving her the freedom to eat the entire supersized tub of buttered popcorn she insisted she wanted goes a lot more towards fueling her learning about her body's fullness than counting out a specific portion or forbidding her from ordering it in the first place.

Another important element of trust, which that little lesson with the bike lock reminds me of: Trust goes both ways. While we need to trust that our daughters can and will *learn* to eat well in time as well as grow into the body that is right for them, they *also* need to know that they can trust us to give them the time, space, and ample opportunity to do it—without criticism, put-downs, disbelief, or personal disappointment. And that means we aren't going to comment on or interfere with each mistake, nor give up on them when they're failing. When we trust them to figure it out, they understand that they are trustworthy, capable, confident, and good—feelings we definitely want to apply to many aspects of their growth that are well beyond their eating.

WHY IS TRUST SO HARD?

Incredible and integral as trust sounds, I'm not going to lie and say it's a snap to pull off. But on those occasions when you do master it, you *and* your children will benefit in amazing ways. For one, you'll be increasing their own eating competence, giving them a good foundation with food and the health and well-being benefits that go along with it. And two, that *not. worrying. about. every. little. thing* is going to feel oh-so-good. Still, I'm not going to sugarcoat it: Trust can be challenging.

Even after working on this chapter for weeks, I ended breakfast this morning by asking my six-year-old, "Are you sure you don't need another bite? You're going to be hungry later." Oops—I overstepped there, didn't I? Helping her get some toast ready, then plating her scrambled eggs and few slices of pear were awesome of me. Calling her back to the table when I noticed she'd eaten less than half of her meal to ask her if she was sure—*not* cool. And that little story about toast that I shared at the start of this book? That was the result of me asking my older daughter one too many times, "Are you sure you're still hungry?" When we ask our kids—even our partners—questions like this, we cause them, even if only for a moment, to question themselves. (And if you want some more proof of how absolutely validating it can feel to not be questioned all the time, see the **Reflection** questions at the end of this chapter for an exercise you can try at home.)

Trusting ourselves and our loved ones with eating is difficult because we are constantly barraged by conflicting messages about food. Threats to our daughter's *eating well-being* or body genius abound in the messages and images we see all the time, every day. They lurk in our subconscious and may surprise us just as much as they shock our kids. Identifying those threats and the sneaky and often paradoxical ways they work is the best way to strengthen our resilience against them. So where does our distrust come from?

WORRY ABOUT WEIGHT AND HEALTH

If we've been living in a larger body ourselves (or have a close loved one who is) we can know firsthand what it feels like to be a victim of weight stigma from being bullied or heckled, to being denied access to medical procedures, to losing job opportunities, to feeling shame when searching for a seat on a plane. If the stakes to our daughter's self-esteem are too high, if the anti-fat bias is coming on too strong, it may feel too risky to test the waters of trust and wait to see how they do with eating.

Even when we're not dieting ourselves or have the good fortune of being in a position to feel indifferent to our place on the weight spectrum or impervious to worries about weight or body shape, we can *still* have strong concerns that certain foods can harm our daughter. We may still take strong action to protect them from those foods by setting limits in the name of good health, by telling her two scoops of ice cream or a particular slice of cake is "too much." Because of our upbringing or the current culture or climate, we may be led to believe that certain foods, such as those high in sugar, are addictive or cause disease. With that in mind, we might view the foods themselves as untrustworthy and worry our daughters will be out of control when eating them.

By the same token, when our child seems to be eating too little of certain foods, we tend to interfere. Every parent has heard another say (or said themselves) at least once, "Don't you think you've had enough of that?" as well as, "Come on, just one more bite." Commonplace as they are, they're still potent problems. Our own fears (conscious or unconscious) about fatness or poor health prompt us to interfere with their knowing and learning without us often even realizing it.

According to research, when parents intervene by trying to control how much bread or broccoli their kids eat, we damage our children's eating competence by weakening their ability to self-regulate.[3] They simply stop listening to their body's intuitive knowing in an effort to please us and worse, if and when they do disobey our limits by eating intuitively to their own individual fullness and satisfaction, they can feel guilty and wrong.

Additionally, if we suggest they stop eating before their body wants or needs them to, we also put them in a mental state of being insecure or unsure that they'll have *enough* food. Research shows that parents who restrict certain foods are more likely to raise kids who become pre-occupied with those foods and overeat or binge on them, not to mention experience a whole host of negative emotions when they do eat them. The impact is similar to what we see with self-restriction in dieting. To be clear, overriding our daughter's *knowing* with eating by telling her to stop not only undermines her self-confidence and self-trust with eating—in all likelihood, over time it will cause her to eat more.

A similar paradoxical phenomenon happens when it comes to pres-suring our kids to eat foods that we consider "good for them" such as vegetables. When we push high-nutrient foods like fruits and veg-etables, we end up decreasing their willingness to try and learn to like those foods on their own. Also important to understand is that even if encouraging our daughters by saying, "Have some more, this is so good for you" or "You need to eat at least half of your vegetables," appears to work in the short term by getting her to give in and take another bite, it's not doing her any favors in the long term. Parents who pressure their children to eat certain foods raise kids who are much less likely to enjoy those very same foods and the effect has been shown to last well into adulthood.[4]

If you're feeling a little guilty here, don't worry. You're not alone. Apparently, the majority of us need to take a collective chill when it comes to interfering with our kids' ability to know how much to eat. By one estimate, 85% of parents admit to trying to get their child to eat more than they wanted to of certain foods, as well as using bribes and praise to do it.[5]

So how can we resist the urge to interfere? By reminding ourselves that if we do resist, we will get much better results! The opposite is also true. Also, if we resist our fears and leave our daughters to their own devices when it comes to how much or how little to eat, they will have a better shot at staying attuned to their inner knowing and eating just the right amounts.[1] If we can resist the urge to pressure them to eat more of the food we believe is healthy and less of the food we believe is not, we increase the odds they will one day learn to like those foods.

Additionally, when weight or health worries crop up during meals, we can help ourselves relax about exactly how many bowls of mac and cheese or how few forkfuls of salad they're eating by reminding ourselves that no *one* meal or habit they have now (or over the last week, month, or year) is enough to define their entire life with food, their body weight, or their overall health. We also need to believe they have the capacity to learn and grow with eating (as opposed to thinking of them as a "picky," or "bad" eater, or a kid who "just loves sweets," or who has "no self-control").

Just like with any other skill they are trying to master, use that growth mindset and remind yourself that it isn't that your daughter "loves sweets too much" or "doesn't eat enough veggies," it is more likely that she hasn't broadened her palate or learned to eat in a balanced way nutritionally speaking *yet*. And, if she seems behind or off-track in these areas, the key is to lean in more with support designed to help increase her *knowing* and lean out when it comes to control, meaning we avoid setting strict limits on amounts she is allowed to or must eat. (I share a tool we can use to support our children's *knowing* without overdoing control later in this chapter.)

FOOD PARENTING CULTURE

Every time we go out to eat together, one of my dearest friends has the infuriating habit of reminding me that her daughter loves salmon. She *loves* it. LOVES. I mean she *really* loves it. Oh, and seaweed and avocado toast. She *loves* those foods, too. L-O-V-E-S. Loves, loves, loves. In my more vulnerable moments, my own daughter's tendency to give fish and greens the side-eye and order the pasta instead makes me twinge just a bit with shame. Despite me knowing better, there are still times when I pick up on the collective concern about children's love of pasta and all that it might imply: *Poor parenting, zero food sophistication, neglect for nutrition, potential for bone disease, cancer, and scurvy to name a few!*

Similar to how diet culture tells us we are wholly responsible for the size and shape of our body, food parenting culture tells us that as parents we are responsible for our child's eating *everything*, from their food likes and dislikes to their ability to self-regulate, and of course, their body weight, shape, and size. We feel guilty if they aren't meeting traditional healthy eating standards, which include high intakes of vegetables, beans, and fish, or if their palate isn't progressing along in variety or sophistication fast enough. And when they don't, we feel compelled to pressure them to change.

So how do we combat those negative feelings about our daughter's eating and resist the urge to interfere by insisting she have a taste of the salmon? We take a few deep breaths. (Is it me, or are deep breaths always the answer?) We can remember our deepest intention for our daughter when it comes to eating. And if that is to have a healthy relationship with food and to be a competent eater then—you guessed it—those are the times when we must lean in extra hard to *trust*. In those moments, we can remind ourselves: *I trust my daughter is doing her best with eating—the best that she is capable of right now. I trust that she will grow normally. I trust that giving her the space to figure out her own likes and dislikes is the best way to support her in becoming a happy, well-adjusted eater. I trust that I am a good mother, a responsive parent, and capable of creating a positive food destiny.*

And then, of course, you do the same thing for yourself by ordering whatever appeals to you instead of what your dearest, I-only-have-your-best-interests-at-heart friend or family member thinks you should be eating. Also consider for a moment that your fellow parenting friends or peers may not be judging your food parenting skills at all—and definitely not as much as you are judging yourself as a parent. In fact, they may be battling some food insecurities of their own. Watching you allow your daughter some freedom with food may even liberate a fellow stressed-out parent do it herself.

OUR OWN HISTORY WITH FOOD

If our mother had an eating disorder, we are at higher risk for developing one ourself.[6] If she was caught in a disordered eating pattern, specifically of dieting and then going overboard on food when her restraint ran out, we are more at risk for developing that pattern too.[7] If she was highly concerned about her appearance, then we as daughters are more likely to share similar concerns. And if she had her own strong weight bias towards others, we are more likely to internalize that too.[8]

So how do mothers' eating issues get passed on through generations? Through a complex web of biological, psychological, and sociocultural factors including genetics, feeding practices, shared eating environments, and their own mother–daughter interpersonal relationship. Some of those factors are transmitted in obvious ways—especially if we've lived through them—while others might leave us scratching our heads and may be more effectively unraveled with the help of a therapist.

Genetics, for example, are considered to be responsible for somewhere between 50-to-80 percent of eating disorders risk, according to researchers.[9] And it's possible that our behaviors around food, such as the way we respond to worries about weight with behaviors like binging and purging, are genetically passed on too. Mothers who restrain themselves around food for some time and then go overboard (a pattern typical of dieting) raise daughters who tend to respond to restriction in the same way and eat in a similar pattern.[7]

As far as feeding, weight-conscious moms who are dieting are more likely to be invested in her daughter's weight and use restrictive feeding to compensate for their concern.[10] If your mom regarded cookies as "empty calories," for example, or started cutting back on starches because of fears that they were linked to anything from diabetes to weight gain to bloating, it makes sense that she might feel more compelled— even obliged—to limit these foods in her children's diets, either by offering them less frequently (if at all) or offering smaller portions.

Relationally speaking, even when they outwardly rebel against them, daughters are naturally inclined to model their mother's behaviors, thoughts, and values, making them a rapt audience for any diet-centric or fat-fearing attitudes and eating habits.[11] That's at least one reason why hearing our mothers talk about their own weight, shape, or size, or be critical of their appearance ups the odds we'll be more prone to body dissatisfaction and more likely to use extreme methods to diet. Lastly, a lack of boundaries between mothers and daughters can facilitate the transmission of eating dysfunction from one to another.[12] (I know! Here's where you may want to have your psychotherapist or counselor on speed-dial, particularly if you're still engaging in these battles with your own mother and in front of your own daughter.)

If you're feeling concerned about how you or your own mother may have already impacted your daughter's eating, please remember this: You are not wholly responsible for your child's function or dysfunction, nor is your mother responsible for yours. A conflux of complicated factors and influences are at play when it comes to how we and our children interact with food and feel about our bodies.

THE TOOL THAT SUPPORTS TRUST

I know what you're thinking. If trust is so challenging, *how am I ever going to do it?* You don't think I'd warn you of the difficulty of something, then just throw you out there into the emotional landmine that is family dinner time without a support system to help you do it, do you? (I wouldn't; I promise!)

Here, I will share with you the tool I use at home with my own girls (and, truth be told, with myself) as well as all the parents I work with. It is called Satter's Division of Responsibility in Feeding (sDOR), also referred to by those that use and teach it as the "trust model." And, I'm guessing it'll come as no surprise that it is a tool designed, developed, and researched by Ellyn Satter, the family feeding guru I refer to throughout this book, as part of the Feeding Dynamics Satter Model (or fdSatter), which is a set of practice and evidence-based principles and recommendations.[13] The concept of trust is the backbone to her work and sDOR is the tool you can use to make it work.

The sDOR is an approach to feeding your family—even yourself—that makes a clear delineation between those two different parts of feeding—the parts we *learn*, practice, and *develop*, and the parts we *know*. Since it takes one of the most stressful parts of feeding—the figuring out how much we should allow or insist that our kids eat—right off our plates (ha!), it's also extremely effective at wiping away the conflict, turmoil, and negative emotions from mealtimes. No more micromanaging those parts of eating that we can only *know*. Without this burden to negotiate, we can relax and enjoy simply eating together, which has been transformative for parents who worry the most about these aspects of feeding.

The sDOR allows parents to offer full permission in a structured, safe way. That is to say, you offer full permission with foods (you can eat as much or as little as you want), but not in a permissive way (you can eat whatever foods you want whenever you want), nor in a neglectful way (you're also in charge of choosing, getting, and preparing those foods for yourself). While we want our girls to be and remain in charge of the *knowing* parts—how much or how little—we also want to offer the multiple types of structure and support to help them do well. The sDOR helps you do that delicate dance between freedom and boundaries that is necessary in so many parts of parenting, guiding you as to exactly where and when to lean in with control, by offering rules and structure, and lean out with control, by giving full permission.

In a nutshell, here's how it works. The sDOR divides responsibilities around mealtime between parents and children. Parents are responsible for **What** foods will be offered, **When** they will be offered, and **Where** they will be offered.

Infants, school-aged kids, adolescents, and teens are responsible for **Whether they will eat or not**, as well as **How much or how little** they will eat. (The *knowing*, as you know.)

At the core of this approach is trust. Parents trust children to handle the *knowing* parts of eating and they show them trust by giving them full permission to eat as much or as little as they like from the foods they have chosen. As parents, we trust our kids to eat as much as they are hungry for, and stop when they are satisfied, and to decide for themselves at any given meal or snack whether they want to eat *at all*. In other words, to eat intuitively as they did in those 26 studies—and presumably to get all those benefits from doing it.

And remember the lesson I learned about trust with the lock? Trust goes both ways. With this approach, children must also trust parents; they must know that they will be offered enjoyable foods at appropriate and predictable intervals. If they trust food will be available regularly—and not just any food—food they are familiar with and can eat without pressure or worry, then they can best do their job of enjoying it intuitively (or in a self-regulated or attuned way). If they're worried food won't be offered or worried it will be something they don't like, or that they will be limited in how much they are allowed to eat (either literally or with the disapproving eye of an adult) then using their *knowing* in the face of that meal will be difficult, if not impossible.

Research on the sDOR is convincing. Parents who use this approach tend to raise children with higher degrees of eating competence—and the benefits that go along with it. That means parents who use the sDOR raise kids who eat better diets (i.e., eat more nutritional variety); feel more joyful and positive about eating; are more trusting and capable with themselves and other people; have better physical self-acceptance; are more active; sleep better and longer; have better medical profiles and lab tests; and do better with feeding their children. By using the sDOR as a tool to guide feeding your family, you'll be giving your daughter the best shot at enjoying food.

While the sDOR is simple to understand, don't underestimate it. It's very effective, yet does require commitment—and a bit of a strong nerve—to be successful at it. In the next section, I share insights into the tendencies that undermine our intentions when it comes to using the sDOR regularly and effectively.

 **Bookmark** Chapter 6: "The Feeding Relationship" in *Secrets of Feeding a Healthy Family* by Ellyn Satter. For readers who are hearing about the sDOR for the first time, I encourage you to learn more about it directly from the aforementioned book, the Ellyn Satter Institute (www. ellynsatterinstitute.org), or by enlisting support from a registered dietitian trained in this model or who use it in combination with other feeding models (particularly if you have a neurodiverse child or one who has experienced significant food trauma or insecurity.)

THAT WON'T WORK FOR MY DAUGHTER!

Many mothers who come to me for nutrition therapy are the savviest of savvy. Many of them have done their parenting homework and know all about the sDOR. I will admit, for as many parents who swear it changed their lives, an equal number say, "It just doesn't work for me." In my experience, I have noticed that many parents who feel frustrated by the fact that everyone else is getting great results except them are often making one of four mistakes.

Misstep #1: Going Permission-Overboard

One of the first mothers who helped make it clear to me just how important a parent's own unresolved history with food could be to their approach to feeding was Jennifer. As she sat in my office and talked to me about her concerns for her daughter, I sensed she was sweet, intelligent, and efficient, as well as deeply vulnerable. While Jennifer had never been diagnosed with an eating disorder herself, during our initial assessment she was astute enough to share with me that she'd been on and off diets for years trying to "fix" the larger body she was in, which her father had disapproved of since she herself was a child. I could see from a growth chart that her daughter, Nora, had been increasing in weight at a rapid rate for the past year. As far as I could tell from Jennifer, both Nora and her brother were thriving in a prestigious and demanding private school, participating in multiple after-school activities, and enjoying time with their friends. Mom seemed to be knocking it out of the park in terms of parenting, juggling her children's busy lives with her own career. The problem was that Jennifer didn't understand the reasons for Nora's recent weight gain, and neither did her pediatrician who recommended she be evaluated by an endocrinologist.

During our session, Jennifer was ambivalent about how she should approach food with both of her children, alternating between offering well-balanced and nutritious meals and multiple opportunities throughout the week to have desserts, sweets, and other treats. She shared that her father was critical of her daughter's weight and recalled a recent incident where at dinner together, her father openly disapproved when Jennifer allowed each of her children to order a dessert. As our visits continued, I sensed how painful it was for Nora to put limits or constraints on her children's eating. While she was doing well with other aspects of feeding and using the sDOR, she still seemed to have trouble not giving in to frequent requests for food outside of the designated eating times, such as saying yes to a stop for ice cream after school or cookies right before bed.

As Jennifer continued to share details of interactions between herself and her father around food, I soon realized that the more critical her father was of her daughter's weight or her way of parenting on any given weekend, the more permissive she would become with her children's eating the following week. Allowing her kids to indulge in what they wanted when they wanted seemed to help Jennifer heal her own years of being restricted and limited. I suspected that she found giving her kids total freedom with food to be very healing.

With some further investigation, I uncovered multiple changes that had occurred in the past year of Nora's life that had likely contributed to the disruption of her growth curve and increase in BMI percentile. (A change in afterschool routine, a decrease in opportunities for activity, increased emotional stress due to her parent's separation and impending divorce, and a new habit of eating two breakfasts in order to socialize more with her friends in the school cafeteria, to name a few. She had also started stopping at the local coffee shop afterschool for a caffeine-containing, high-calorie drink, which subsequently kept her up well past bedtime and left her looking for extra late-night snacks for energy not to mention exhausted the following day.) What was most interesting, however, was how her grandfather's increasing influence had reignited Jennifer's negative feelings about her own weight and, ultimately, shifter her willingness to stick to the sDOR as well as her commitment to intuitive eating.

Many mothers who have recovered from dieting or lifelong restriction use intuitive eating, as I did and as I suspect Jennifer did, to get to a good place with food. If we have been dieting or limiting for a long time, it allows us to let go of many of our deceptively harmful eating inhibitions. With our newfound freedom, it makes sense that we want to hand over full permission to our daughters, too. It also makes sense that if we have had a lot of childhood trauma around eating, whether it was self-inflicted through our own dieting, restriction put on us by our parents, or restriction put on us because of circumstances beyond our own or our parents' control (such as not having access to food or enough food regularly), then enforcing limits can be extra emotional and hard. It can feel easier—even liberating—to allow a child to have full control over every single aspect of eating.

Intuitive eating can help us as chronic dieters and our children return or stay in touch with our own skills of internal regulation. However, there is a very important difference between intuitive eating and the sDOR, and that difference is *structure*.

The Fix: Focusing on Structure. Nora had the full permission part of eating down pat, which was a feat in and of itself, given how much pressure there is to do just the opposite. The part of her healthy feeding approach that she was missing was what Satter calls *discipline*. Since discipline sounds scary to me as a former dieter, we can also call it structure. While limits on types and amounts of food aren't necessary (or even recommended) with intuitive eating, guiding our children—even our own eating—with some structure and the form of limits around time and place is an important key to healthy eating.

What Nora was missing was constraints, or structure, around her children's eating. Here are the benefits of using structure, such as deciding on the *time* and *place* of your kids' eating ahead of time. Having a solid structure to meals and snacks will help your daughter:

- **Get better at intuitive eating**. Letting time—but not too much—pass between meals and snacks help you and your daughter arrive to the table hungry but not starving, making it easier to stay calm and listen to internal cues. Knowing there's a consistency and predictability in when we will eat can help those of us who eat too much or tend to be overly focused on and concerned about food.

- **Decrease overeating.** Having meals and snacks at scheduled times reassures them that more food is coming and encourages us to enjoy only what we need to feel satisfied.

- **Decrease pickiness and fussiness about foods**. When we are hungry, we are more likely to try something new or eat something despite it not being our favorite food. If we sit to eat and we're not particularly hungry, we tend to be more selective and search harder for something on the table (or in your cupboards) that really appeals to us. That's one reason why kids tend to pressure us to cater to their likes.

- **Make mealtimes more pleasant.** When kids can easily predict when meals and snacks will be, they come to them feeling much happier and less anxious or stressed about their eating.

- **Keep caregivers sane.** (This one's not scientifically proven, but I can vouch for it anecdotally!) If you have a set schedule that's known to you AND your daughter, you've set healthy boundaries around the kitchen and eating. That means you're no longer constantly catering to requests for food. Nor are you worrying about whether your child ate enough. You remind yourself that she will have an opportunity to eat again at the next meal.

Misstep #2: Not Giving Enough Permission

Sometimes when pediatric dietitians teach the sDOR and cooperative, caring, and responsive parents struggle to get results, the RD will ask mom or dad to film a few meals. Why would a dietitian request a video of your family eating? Because feeding dynamics are complex. Even when we have the best intention to trust our child to eat intuitively, believing that our children will learn to stop when they've had enough, as long as they are consistently given permission to do it, can still feel scary. Many of us might think we're letting go all the way when it comes to trying to curb their eating, when in fact we may still be sending subtle messages that we want them to stop. A parent might quickly clear a plate at the very first indication that the child has slowed with eating, prompt them to drink more water, or overemphasize vegetables by plating large amounts while cooking limited amounts of starch.

The Fix: Remembering the Paradox. For those of us who struggle with permission, or who find it hard to relax, bite our tongue, and remain impassioned as we watch our daughter reach for her fourth helping of extra creamy mac and cheese or listen as she requests some Oreos as a snack between school and soccer, consider a concept I use to calm myself when I'm feeling the impulse to interfere with "I think that's enough bread" or "If you want extra, why don't you try these strawberries before you have any more cookies?" The concept is this: Permission with food has a paradox built in.

The more permission we allow ourselves and our children with highly desirable foods, the more relaxed and in control we and our kids feel in the face of it. The less permission we allow ourselves or our children with food, the more we tend to eat and the more out-of-control—or disconnected from our inner knowing—we are when eating.

Misstep #3: Forgetting That Responsibilities Change with Age

The division of responsibility is not static. It is meant to flex and change over time, with the handing of responsibilities from child to caregiver, then back again to child. Once you understand this concept, you'll be better able to navigate the questions that come up such as, "Shouldn't she be making her own lunch?" And "But I thought only parents decide *what's* for dinner?"

During infancy, a baby is in charge of many aspects of eating, including where, when, and how much or how little. You don't tell a four-month-old to wait until lunchtime. And, yes, I remember the days of pulling off the highway to nurse a screaming infant. At that point, you are essentially only in charge of what (breastmilk or formula) and she's in charge of everything else.

However, once your child's tummy can hold more food, you start to gradually take over the responsibilities of deciding time and place, for example designating set times for snacks and meals. She remains in charge of the knowing or body-led parts of eating, such as how much or how little or whether or not she will eat at all. From there, the sDOR recommends a gradual shifting of responsibilities to kids as they grow, such as deciding what and when to eat.

The Fix: Learning When to Hand Off What. Remember, it's a hand-off of your feeding responsibilities, one by one by one from highchair to college. Here's how it breaks down based on Satter. When your daughter was an infant, it's pretty clear that you decided what to feed (breastmilk or formula) and she decided everything else, when, where, whether, how much or how little. As she started eating solids, you still decided the what in terms of what you'd offer (peas or avocado, applesauce or egg, for example) and gradually started taking more control of where and when. She decided whether or how much. As she starts getting to be school age, the when and where become less and less in her control and are fully defined by you (and in some cases outside things such as school), while she remains in charge of whether and how much. Elementary school and middle school is where some shifts start to happen. Some kids start to be interested in and help with food preparation, though parents should still be supervising them and deciding on the what, when, and where of meals. For example, if they are putting together a sandwich for lunch, parents should provide guidance as to what—pointing out, for example, that a peanut butter and jelly sandwich, a glass of milk, and an apple constitute a balanced plate as opposed to making an entire meal a bag of chips.

Older adolescents, such as those in middle school, may have more autonomy with when and where, and can be in charge of the what for at least some meals and snacks. Lunch may be left up to a sixth-grader completely, if she can now buy lunch at school. (You can also gradually shift responsibility in even small increments here, by allowing her to buy lunch one day per week then increasing it in a few months or the next academic year. Or if you're still packing a lunch, you might let her do it herself once weekly, including allowing her to decide *what* it will be.) This is a great time to practice and give your daughter a chance to experiment with food choices and learn on her own. During adolescence, parents should be in charge of the what, when, and where for the majority of meals, however. High schoolers have increasing autonomy with the *what* and *when*, deciding on their own if they need an extra snack after school, or *what* and *when* they will have dinner, when they are away from their parents for longer periods on the weekends or evenings. Throughout all of these years, parents should still be setting the pace and tone of feeding, providing the guidance and overall structure needed by keeping up with shared meal times.[14]

Feeling like things are a little off in your home with regard to eating? You can figure out what might be off in terms of responsibilities between you and your daughter by making a quick spreadsheet-like list. In a column on the left going down, write each meal and snack (example, breakfast, lunch, snack, dinner) based on your daughter's current eating schedule. Then across the top make three columns labeled "what," "when," and "where." For each box you create, check those she's currently responsible for. Then think about which, if any, responsibilities you'd like to transfer to your child or have your child transfer to you based on the above guidance on age.

Ultimately, the goal is to have all those boxes checked by the time she does live on her own and becomes fully responsible for her own feeding.

Misstep #4: Pushing Aside Your Mom Instincts Completely

The sDOR is a guide, a roadmap to give us direction when "winging it" with family feeding is too hard or problematic. Understanding how and why it works as well as what it solving for is key when it comes to making it work for your family. As with all parenting advice, I don't recommend that you follow it so rigidly that it causes you to silence your own best instincts or prevents you from being tuned in to and responsive to your child's unique needs. You know your daughter best. If there are times when deviating from the model are in her best interests (say, for example, giving into an occasional before-bed request for food from a child who you feels needs it due to hunger or other reasons), I hope you will feel the freedom to do it.

If you're struggling with the sDOR, get support. Work with a pediatrician, registered dietitian, or therapist who has been trained by the Satter Institute, someone who fully understands the nuances of this approach—as well as responsible deviations from it—and can help you identify what might be keeping it from working for you.

THE TRUST LITMUS TEST

Since trust is hard, questions around it abound. Even after a parent has been using the sDOR for months or a colleague has been studying and teaching the model for years, questions come up. The good news? There's an easy way to answer them.

I call it the "trust litmus test" in my practice.

When parents come to me and ask, "Is it okay to just serve less bread?" or "Don't you think I should just stop buying chips?" I tell them to give those questions the Trust Litmus Test. Ask yourself, *Is this leading with trust or control?*

When you lead with *control*, even when you feel it's in their best interests or you're trying to protect them (or yourself) from some outcome with food, you're going to get into some trouble. Especially if that control is doubling as restriction or restraint. If a rule is about *trust and enjoyment*, then it is positive and helpful. If a rule is about *control and avoidance*, then it is likely harming you or your child.

When my girls ask me if they can have Girl Scout cookies at snack time and I decide to take just two chocolate-covered discs out of the box—one for each of them—then toss the rest in the bottom of the garbage when they're not looking, am I operating from a place of trust or control? I ask myself, Am I giving them an opportunity to enjoy the cookies without worry about when they'll ever get them again? Or to learn how many they like to eat? Or am I stealing that choice by putting in a hard stop before they ever get the chance to make the mistake of having the feeling for themselves of eating "one too many"? Control has the allure of making me feel safer as a parent and feeder, but it's doing nothing for my daughters as eaters except making them feel deprived and unsure about their ability to indulge in pleasurable food on their own. It's important for us to trust not just the fact that our daughters can be trusted with knowing how much to eat, but also their ability to learn. When we fully trust that they will, we can give them the time and space to make the mistakes they need to make, in order to grow into a competent eater.

• •

When we tell our daughters that they've had enough and to stop eating, we are also telling them to distrust messages from their body, particularly from their hunger and appetite. When we tell our daughters that they have not eaten enough, we are essentially telling them that their sense of satiation is not to be trusted. And, while I don't have any science on this part, I believe that on a deeper level, we risk setting them up to distrust many other aspects of their bodily experiences. You may already sense how destructive this can be on many other parts of her bodily experiences. (What other body sensations, for example, should they trust or not trust? That tightness in the chest they get when a stranger pulls up next to them, or a conversation with a friend that feels off, or that butterflies-in-the-stomach feeling they get just before they're about to try something that may be unsafe?)

IFM Touchstone: *Trust*

What area of eating do you trust your daughter with the least? Which area do you think she distrusts you the most? What is one small action you can take to help build trust in one of these areas? For example, *I intend to avoid commenting on how much my daughter is eating* or *I intend to create a clear and realistic meal schedule for each day of the week.*

Trusting our daughters to learn to grow into competent eaters is crucial. If we don't trust them and encourage them to tune into their own body for information about hunger and fullness, we teach them they cannot trust themselves and we set them up for a lifetime of feeling unsure about food and wondering when and if it's okay to eat. Self-trust is vital if we're going to be full, whole beings. If we don't trust the signals we get from within, we live in constant conflict. And if we send our daughters the message that we can't trust them with something as fundamental as eating, then we risk teaching them that at their very core they aren't trustworthy. The good news is, since trust is fundamental to our eating, we are born fundamentally good at it.

REFLECTIONS FOR TRUST

- *Do you trust your daughter to eat as much or as little as she wants and her body needs?*

- *What do you think your daughter feels when it comes to being trusted with food and eating? Does she feel she is trusted—or not trusted?*

- *If you are struggling with trust and food, what is your fear? What do you believe will happen if you started trusting your daughter to eat as little or as much as she needs?*

- *What might be the consequence of not trusting her with food? How might it impact her relationship with food or her eating habits in the future?*

- *What might be the benefit of increasing trust with food? How might it impact her relationship with food or her eating habits in the future?*

- *When we respond to our daughter with questions, it can make her second guess herself or feel as though she is being challenged To help her feel more trusted and confident, try this: avoid stating anything as a question for a set time period of, say, 20 minutes. Instead, respond by restating what you've heard her say. This reflexive gesture will signal that to her that she's been heard—and whatever she's saying or feeling is okay.*

CHAPTER SEVEN
ACCEPTANCE

"I will not teach or love or show you anything perfectly,
but I will let you see me, and I will always hold sacred the
gift of seeing you. **Truly, deeply, seeing you**."

—*Brene Brown, The Wholehearted Parenting Manifesto, Daring Greatly*

THE PARENTING PROWESS I DEMONSTRATED ON THE MORNING of my daughter's eighth birthday was cringeworthy, exactly the kind of stuff that makes you know that your child will one day be in therapy, for sure.

I was standing in my kitchen, studying a picture on Pinterest while doing my best to put the finishing touches on her "Happy Birthdae Harry" cake, worrying about what the other parents might think about the box cake covered in mile-high frosting that I'd be offering their children, when I heard her coming down the stairs. She was wearing a fuchsia dress with a miniature flower print on the bottom half that reminded me of wallpaper you'd see in a New England bed and breakfast in the 80s. Her hair was up in a high pony, and she was wearing two of her favorite accessories—a shiny, maroon-and-yellow Gryffindor necktie and a plastic, rainbow-colored choker with a unicorn charm. She was smiling brightly, aware of nothing but the cake.

Did I say, "Happy Birthday!" and then acknowledge the bright positives of the situation, such as the fact that she had gotten herself dressed all on her own, even brushed her hair and chosen some accessories without nary a parent asking? (A skill we'd been working on for months, I might add.) Or that I'd nearly pulled off the exact cake she requested in time for her party. Nope—I didn't.

Unfortunately, I went with, "Are you *sure* you want to wear *that* today? What happened to that adorable blue dress we just bought you?"

My daughter's sweet, expectant smile faded.

I closed my eyes and pressed into my better self. If my intention was to raise my girls to care less about how other people think they look and stay focused on who they *are* and how they *feel*, and if my want was for them to be wholly accepting of themselves, including their tastes in clothing and food, then I'd failed on two accounts and needed to remedy the situation immediately!

"I'm so sorry, sweetie! What I meant to say is that... I'm so happy you chose the dress you like the best!" And if I ever get invited to one of those therapy sessions, I will explain that acceptance was something I certainly wasn't winning at, but had earnestly been working on.

ACCEPTANCE ACCELERATES GROWTH

As imperfect as my attempts at acceptance might be, I've discovered that mastering this particular aspect of parenting pays massive dividends. Not only does it have the potential to enhance my relationship with my daughter and increase our connection, it also helps her have an improved relationship with herself.

Girls who experience more acceptance from their parents enjoy better overall well-being, including protection from depression, anxiety, and even more longevity.[1] When we offer our daughters our own acceptance, as well as offer them empathy for what they perceive as shortcomings, flaws, or imperfections, their own self-acceptance grows. When she is more accepting of herself just as she is, she can feel more at home in the world, more at peace, more whole, grounded, stable, and true.

Helping our daughters to cultivate self-acceptance in one area (for example, going easy on themselves despite the fact that math or soccer doesn't come naturally to them) can also help them be more accepting of themselves in other areas of their lives where they may perceive themselves to be flawed (body size or looks, academic or athletic ability). Helping girls cultivate an attitude of self-acceptance has the power to extend well beyond issues with eating or body or physical ability. Research shows that those of us who are self-accepting are more likely to enjoy increased emotional resilience and physical health throughout life.[2]

When we—and our girls—can embody self-compassion and acceptance, we bounce back from setbacks more quickly because we take them in stride. When we can take setbacks in stride, we are more likely to persevere through failures and misunderstandings. These skills are important for a successful life, because in what world will our daughter ever live where she *doesn't* make mistakes or experience setbacks? In what world will she not fall short or fail to live up to at least some ideals? None. Being accepting of that fact right from the beginning seems quite necessary indeed.

Acceptance doesn't mean we suddenly have to sign off on everything we don't like about ourselves, our daughters, our relationships, or our past. It means we accept what is without judgment. Acceptance is more about self-awareness than it is about giving up on what we care about. And, ironically, psychologists point out that it's an important step towards making change in the future, so if you've got concerns about yourself, your daughter, or your relationship, accepting what is as well as how you feel about it is a good place to start.

Acceptance and self-acceptance are different than self-esteem. Self-esteem is feeling value based on our accomplishments and behaviors, while self-acceptance is feeling valued unconditionally. Offering a lot of praise over a thing done well or outcomes is much different—and the positive effects don't last as long—than offering praise for effort regardless of the outcome. The feeling of value and worthiness one gets through self-acceptance lasts throughout ups and downs and increases our resilience, whereas the ego boost we get from accomplishments is more vulnerable to just fading away.

In my mind, the benefits of supporting our daughters in increasing their own self-compassion and self-acceptance can improve their potential exponentially.

My daughter was eight years old. The fact that she cared more about looking like JoJo Siwa than a Gap ad and would rather eat a box cake with an inch of pink frosting than the one sourced from fresh ingredients picked up from the farmer's market is absolutely and reassuringly developmentally normal, as well as harmless. Let's face it: nothing tragic has ever come out of a bit of bad taste in clothing. And despite what many health experts may have us believe, nothing tragic ever came to a child who preferred a birthday cake sweetened with sugar and decorated with processed, store-bought toppings rather than organic fruit compote and gluten-free flour, either. My questioning her choices, on the other hand, could cause plenty of emotional grief.

What my eight-year-old needed in that moment was not my judgment, criticism, disapproval, or questions, but my wholehearted *acceptance*. I needed to get control of my own emotions and check them against the reality of the situation, as well as remember my intention to prioritize my daughter's well-being over everything else.

ACCEPTANCE AIN'T ALWAYS EASY

One thing I've learned as a nutrition therapist—and, I suppose as a human—is that just because someone is rock solid about wanting to change a behavior, that doesn't necessarily mean it will be easy to do.

So I've been digging deep to figure out why offering our kids unconditional acceptance feels tough. Turns out, a lot of things are at play including natural approaches to parenting; unconscious attitudes about foods; ineffective communication styles; the parenting habits and expectations we learned from our own parents; and, not surprising, our tendency to have a tough time being accepting of ourselves. With a little insight into each, acceptance becomes a lot easier to master.

DISAPPROVAL IS OUR DEFAULT REACTION

It's not just you; it's a parenting thing. Despite the seemingly obvious association between disapproval and dysfunction, often even the most conscientious of parents can't help disapproving of at least some of their child's behaviors and choices, particularly around food. Many of us feel almost obliged to sigh heavily when our child reaches for a second slice of cake at a birthday party, or roll our eyes if we hear them say they'd love to get lunch at McDonald's. Along with our associations between fast food and heart disease or sugar and diabetes, we may unconsciously feel that admonishing our daughter for her food preference is what we must do to protect her. Food isn't the only place parents feel compelled to disapprove. In fact, it's the *modus operandi* and default reaction behind many aspects of other aspects of parenting, and there's often a tendency to rely on it as a strategy for changing what we feel is unsafe or unwell in our kids.

"Most people have been brought up to believe that if you accept a child, [she] will remain just the way [she] is; that the best way to help a child become something better in the future is to tell [her] what you *don't* accept about him now," explains communication expert and three-time Nobel Peace Prize winning psychologist Thomas Gordon, Ph.D., (pronouns changed). "Therefore, most parents rely heavily on the language of *unacceptance* in rearing children, believing this is the best way to help them."

The problem? As you probably can guess, disapproval doesn't work. In fact, it triggers shame and hurt. And it's probably no surprise that kids who experience more rejection, criticism, and disapproval from their parents are more likely to be depressed, anxious, and irritable.[3] (In other words, I *really* needed to lighten up about the dress, the cake, and just about everything else.)

Our acceptance, on the other hand, can help our daughters bloom. "Acceptance is like the fertile soil that permits a tiny seed to develop into the lovely flower it is capable of becoming. The soil only *enables* the seed to become the flower. It *releases* the capacity of the seed to grow, but the capacity is entirely within the seed. As with the seed, a child contains entirely within [her] organism the capacity to develop. Acceptance is like the soil—it merely enables the child to actualize [her] potential," explains Gordon.

Just like taste in clothing, we all have our own personal eating style. You may prefer heavy foods or lighter ones. You might like your chili jalapeno level spicy, or you might not like chili at all. You might eat fast, or you might eat slow. You might like your soup lukewarm or steaming hot. You might like to eat breakfast like a queen and dinner like a pauper, or the other way around. You may eat to live or live to eat. (I'm of the live to eat ilk, how about you?). Some of us have small appetites and low hunger, and some of us have big ones. (I fall in the latter camp with this one, too!)

Perhaps because we mistakenly think our kids' eating style is in our control (much like how I felt about my daughter's clothing style), we seem to feel obligated to fix or correct the tastes and styles we don't like. In contrast, we are very accepting of the food preferences and eating styles of the adults in our life. The fact that your best girlfriend won't eat anything with cilantro, or that your cousin refuses to touch a plate if it's also touched a tomato? Well, those things are just *them*. When our own kids tell us they don't like foods spicy, many of us feel compelled to insist that they *just try it* or that when it comes to what they like, they're just plain wrong.

Just like we want to avoid rejection of our daughter on a personal level, we want to avoid rejecting her on many microlevels of her eating, too. While disapproving of her food choices may seem like an effective way to help her avoid being a "bad" eater, it isn't. Refusing or rejecting her food preferences is totally unnecessary, in terms of protecting her health, and could be damaging.

For some kids, parental disapproval may be as effective and have the same results as overt food restriction, meaning that while your daughter might take fewer french fries or limit herself to just one cookie, she's also more likely to overeat those foods in the future. Even if this technique does stop her from eating what you feel is unhealthy for the time being, over the long term she may end up eating more. Our acceptance is what can truly help her progress with her eating.

If disapproval feels like it's part of your parenting style and you want to let it go, you can start by noticing patterns you might have picked up from your own childhood. While one-on-one therapy is the best way to do this, you can get started in releasing patterns by getting curious about how you were parented around food using questions in the **Reflections** section of this chapter.

ACCEPTANCE ISN'T ABOUT GREENLIGHTING EVERYTHING

Does acceptance mean we are okay with everything our child does? Nope! You can still have strong boundaries with your daughter, as well as want things to improve. However, saying no to something or wanting to work towards a different outcome is very different from disapproving of where your daughter is with a skill, habit, or behavior.

Disapproval triggers guilt, remorse, and embarrassment. Saying no to something—with a good, clear reason for it—doesn't. It may frustrate her, but it won't trigger shame. If we disapprove of our daughter crossing the street without looking by shaking our head in disgust or giving her a stern look as she attempts to do it, she will probably feel shame. Think about that reaction versus how she might feel if, in the same situation, you instead put your arm out in front of her and said firmly, "No. That is dangerous. We need to look both ways first," without any criticism at all.

Disapproving of "unhealthy" eating habits may seem like a good way to help our daughters eat better; however, as we learned in the chapter on trust, it is more likely to trigger internal conflict, leaving our girls with negative feelings like self-doubt and shame about eating. That doesn't mean we can't say, "No, we are not having ice cream for dinner," we just support our daughters better if we are a little less impassioned, critical, and disparaging, and a little more matter-of-fact when we do it.

The sDOR is a great strategy that can help us be more neutral and accepting about our child's eating, since it includes a set of clear boundaries and constraints that we, as parents and leaders, have set. When the rules are clear—such as no grabbing food from the pantry between meals or eating in whatever room you want—we can be a lot less emotional about enforcing them. It's not a criticism to say "Stop grabbing a snack before dinner" when you can point out that it's a firm family rule you have put in place for a reason. And, of course, we need to be clear that those rules are never about weight control, but instead about supporting overall well-being and the more practical parts of eating, such as "I want you to be hungry when it's time for dinner."

ACCEPTANCE IS MORE THAN A MINDSET

So, here's the thing: Setting an intention to be accepting towards our daughter's eating is glorious, valiant, and totally necessary. However, when it comes to protecting them from a whole host of food-related dysfunction, it's only the first step.

Acceptance is more than a mindset, an attitude, or a feeling, explains Gordon. Acceptance is an act you commit daily and "must be actively communicated or demonstrated," he clarifies. So how do we actively communicate acceptance? With the words and tone we use when we talk about food, and with the rules and boundaries we have around eating.

Communicating Acceptance with Words. A few years into my practice, I noticed a pattern. No matter how much parents and I would discuss positive feeding practices, which foods to offer, and the concept of balancing permission with structured meals, inevitably a parent would end the session by asking me some version of, "Okay. So what should I *say?*" It was as if, just at the moment they were about to put on their coats to leave, they wanted to boil down all the techniques and approaches we had talked about into a few delicate words.

First of all, I maintain that whenever possible, it's best to say nothing. We don't need to try to talk our children into trying foods or eating specific amounts. And as I've mentioned in an earlier chapter, unless they ask and are interested, providing a lot of information about nutritional qualities of foods isn't recommended. Making good choices about what you offer and then being indifferent to their decision to eat them is the approach that'll get you the best results.

Staying mum on the topic of food all together isn't always realistic or possible, however. So, with this reality in mind, I started digging around in the research to answer the question *Do the words parents use to talk about food impact their children's eating?* I learned that, yes, they do. And it's not only what parents say—it's *how* we say it that matters.

We've already discussed that parents who avoid linking weight and food tend to raise kids who are more protected from disordered eating. And that there's a benefit to avoiding being critical or judgmental towards our own eating by saying things such as, "I really shouldn't be eating this" or "this is too fattening" in front of our kids. Self-criticism, remember, harms you just as much as an impressionable girl who hears it.

It's also best to avoid words like "bad," "junk," and "unhealthy" when it comes to talking about foods and drinks. Labeling certain foods as evil triggers feelings of guilt, low self-esteem, and shame in the people who eat them. Your food disapprovals can be especially harmful if you're referring to something your daughter eats often or really enjoys. Another reason to avoid name-calling when it comes to food: When we do this, we inadvertently teach our daughters to be critical of others who eat them as "wrong," "bad," or deserving of shame, too. It's important to keep our attitudes positive and open as opposed to fearful and critical, which can create internalized conflict about eating. When talking about food with your daughter, emphasize function and enjoyment and keep it factual, not emotional. For example, "Our body uses pasta (or carbohydrates) for energy, to help us move or think quickly." Talk like this highlights the function of food. "This soup is so creamy and delicious," highlights pleasure, and "These cookies are based on a recipe from Brazil" is factual.

As you will learn in Chapter 8, all foods provide nourishment. Sure, we may choose to offer our kids certain foods over others, and that's not a problem. It's the overt disapproval and judgment of foods and our lack of acceptance if we, our daughters, or others enjoy them that causes the problem.

Communicating Acceptance with Tone. Remember that story I shared at the start of this book, the one with myself, my daughter, and the extra slice of toast? I realized that it didn't matter how often I said yes to food, what mattered was whether I was actively communicating acceptance. And clearly, the shame in her voice said I wasn't. What revealed my deeper misgivings wasn't a lack of permission, it was the subtle disapproval evident in my tone.

Perhaps it didn't matter that I never talked about calories, or good foods and bad foods, or dieting, or weight. The toast incident was evidence that I had somehow still managed to unconsciously transmit my own deeply buried ambivalence—disapproval even—of my daughter's appetite, her hunger, and her *knowing*.

To actively communicate an attitude of acceptance, we must be *direct* and *positive* when it comes to giving instructions or guidance about eating food, as well as handling requests and rejections of food. When you start to listen, you might notice that food comments are often indirect. And depending on our underlying attitudes or fears, they can be negative, too. Saying, "Do you want another one?" with an inviting smile is different from asking "Do you want *another* one?" as if it is an accusation.

When talking to kids about food, be gentle, kind, and guiding—while remaining concrete and clear. Children are more likely to listen to direction when they feel respected and supported, and when they clearly understand your request. They are less likely to comply with requests that are critical, shaming, or coercing. Worse? Such comments are known to lower self-esteem and cause overeating. For example,

"Sweetheart, take one cookie only so there is enough for everyone," works much better than, "Please stop. You're always asking for sweets."

SELF-ACCEPTANCE IS THE MOTHER OF ACCEPTANCE

Last night, as I walked towards my daughter's bedroom, I heard a sound that made me stop just short of the door. She was humming a song. I leaned against the wall to steady myself against a sudden wave of heat, love, and swirling awe. I was reminded, as I am many times throughout the day, that my daughter is a wonderous being, her very own miracle. She's tender, dreamy, vulnerable, and stoic all at once, and, in so many exceptional ways, nothing like me at all.

What's baffled me is this: If I can so often feel such reverence for my daughters, then why at other moments can I also be so critical and frustrated, cutting, and filled with disapproval? How can I adore so much of each of my girls' being, yet the preference for something as inconsequential as the pink dress, her request for extra toast, or love of super sugary cake is unacceptable?

What I have come to realize is this: I can't give away something I don't have.

A hard look at myself makes it clear that the moments when I've been quick to criticize, judge, or respond in a way that's brash and un-filtered towards my daughters, it's seemed always to be about something related to their appearance or a project about their weight. (Cringy, I know! But I'm being honest.) In case you haven't already noticed a theme here, those are the same things I've struggled to accept about myself. And with that, I'm doing exactly what has been done to every other young woman in this world, which is to objectify her, to *see* her more than *know* her, and to transmit my own self-criticisms onto her.

With some self-awareness, however, I'm beginning to shift the tide. When my disapproval wells up (or, gulp, goes as far as to slip out be-cause, yes, it still does), I recognize it and remind myself of its harm.

I reconfirm my deepest intention to see her for who she is, to accept her, to lead with trust instead of control, and to stop worrying about the neatness, cuteness, performance, or perfectness of her looks or her weight. If the critical voice is about food, I recommit to my own IFM

I embrace self-acceptance as a parent—I am flawed but trying to do better, after all—and model for her the gift of self-acceptance. I want to give her the confidence to know that her appetite, and style, and weight are hers and hers alone. So are her beliefs, her inner strengths, her intelligence, passions, and even her limits. They are all her. When it comes to her value, the only thing that matters is not how she is seen, but who she *is*. When we offer ourselves self-compassion with the challenging job at hand, we are paving the way for her own self-acceptance should she ever slip up when it comes to meeting her personal goals and also staying true to her own deepest intentions.

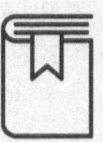

Bookmark: *The Body is Not an Apology* by Sonya Renee Taylor. If you want powerful inspiration (and a gameplan) to help you work on your own self-acceptance, then who better than an author who identifies as being impacted by multiple systems of oppression—yet embodies radical self-love despite it—to help you?

ACCEPTANCE & OUR 'TUDE TOWARD FOOD

Our attitude towards food fuels our approval or disapproval of just about everything that has to do with eating. Once we understand that communicating an attitude of acceptance towards our daughter's eating habits and food choices is a strategy that can help her develop and improve her eating skills, then making sure we are operating from a calm and pleasant place (as opposed to a fearful, critical one) becomes essential. When we understand our attitude towards food, we can create a more positive experience with eating and have less conflict around food, both within ourselves and between ourselves and our daughters. Additionally, some research suggests that when we feel better about what we're eating, we have better digestion and absorb more nutrients, which means having a positive attitude about food can make meals easier on your tummy and even more nourishing!

What are our attitudes towards food and where do they come from? Our eating attitudes are what we think, feel, and believe about food and eating styles. Our eating attitudes dominate our priorities and behaviors when it comes to choosing and eating foods. They can be both subtle and overt, conscious and unconscious, shared and individualized, and positive and negative.

Our attitudes towards foods are formed from the time we are young and continue to be influenced daily. Our upbringing, of course, has had a huge impact on how we think and feel about specific foods and ways of eating. Whether they realized it or not, our parents or other people who fed us were constantly persuading us to like certain foods and favor certain preparation styles and avoid others based on a whole host of complicated factors including their own culture, upbringing, and values.

For example, in my mother's family there's a shared belief that homemade meals are the most precious and valued because of the time, attention, and care that goes into preparing them. Meals include recipes passed down through generations. Making sure that foods are prepared in the traditional ways using traditional ingredients is important, and a shared belief not just among our family but also the larger Italian culture. In another family, the attitude towards homemade food might be quite different—perhaps eating out is considered more respected than eating at home because it requires less time or is done by a professional, such as a chef. Or perhaps eating together isn't prioritized at all.

Our environment also shapes our attitudes; is food available, affordable, and consistently so? How do people around us feel about growing food versus buying it? Is eating organic or local important, or is imported food regarded as special?

In addition to our upbringing, our eating attitudes are formed based on our own experiences as well as by persuasion. In the chapter on influence, we learned how the larger culture persuades us towards certain attitudes about foods and styles of eating. If we've been persuaded by diet or health culture to adopt a "thinner is better/healthier" perspective, then we are more swayed by celebrities, media, podcasters, book authors, and bloggers to have attitudes of disdain, distrust, and fear towards foods that are high in sugar, high in fat, or highly palatable (lest we might enjoy them "too much"). We start to shape our attitudes towards foods, food groups, food brands, and food preparation styles based on whatever they decide to tell or sell us.

Our attitudes can be mutable and may change. Say, for example, our first experience of a jalapeño was that it burned our tastebuds terribly, so we regard it negatively with an attitude of contempt and fear. Then, upon reading in a health magazine that capsaicin—a compound found in jalapeños—speeds up metabolism and burns fat, you may start to regard jalapeños with interest and curiosity. Coconut oil, for example, may have been something you felt indifferent towards because of a lack of experience with it or even apprehension because you knew it was high in saturated fats. Then you read an article on a well-known website that said coconut oil can help speed up fat loss, improve skin texture, and even boost your memory. Those are some pretty persuasive claims, enough to shift your attitude towards this product when you see it on a supermarket shelf.

Our attitudes are often nuanced, as well. For example, you had the pleasurable experience of eating a creamy scoop of hazelnut gelato on a special trip to Italy with your family as a child. Your attitude toward that food might be one of pleasure, joy, affection, and even playfulness. Then you read in a book that eating white sugar—such as the kind that's in your favorite cool treat—causes weight gain and is addictive. Now you've been persuaded to have an attitude of distrust and disdain for this food. We don't forget about those earlier experiences, nor do we drop our attitudes about them, we just couple them up with the negative ones we've been persuaded to adopt and live in a state of emotional tug-of-war.

In the United States, our collective attitudes towards eating are quite conflicting. In general, we share the belief that eating is crucial to good health. Yet, we rarely prioritize eating.

For example, time spent planning, preparing, and eating meals and snacks is undervalued, and therefore the time we devote to them is expected to be limited. We have an attitude that it's our moral duty to eat well, yet also believe that time spent eating is indulgent and therefore ends up being limited. We grab food on the go or skip meals altogether. We expect our children to do well with a 20-minute break for lunch during school or munch on snacks in our cars as we move from activity to activity. We often eat while scrolling through our phones, tidying up the kitchen, answering emails, or sometimes while working on several of these tasks in between sips and bites all at once.

We also share the belief that food is medicine and a health elixir. Yet, we approach many foods with fear, avoidance, and a less-is-more attitude. Delicious foods pose a threat and healthy foods feel obligatory. With this in mind, we approach meal planning and eating (food shopping or even ordering off a menu) with self-doubt, worry, and insecurity. This doesn't bode well for those of us who need to plan, prepare, and eat multiple times a day, every single day, which is just about everyone!

Thinking about your own attitudes about foods and eating can help you understand why you feel conflicted about your own food or your daughter's choices of foods or style of eating. Your daughter might have a positive attitude towards a donut, for example, because it tastes delicious, is colorful and playful, and she once ate one with her favorite uncle after a soccer game. On the other hand, if your attitude toward donuts is one of fear because you've been persuaded to think sugar is highly addictive, or perhaps because you know donuts are high calorie and you've noticed her shorts are getting tight, there's bound to be a lot of conflict, not only internally, but between the two of you. While she might have a positive experience eating the donut, you might feel a lot of shame and guilt from letting her.

When we leave our attitudes towards food unexamined, they fester, persist, and even intensify. Unexamined feelings dominate us, causing us to act impulsively and without understanding. When we notice our feelings, respect them, and bring them out into the open, they lose their power. If we have the courage to do this regularly, over time, they may even disintegrate completely. Sometimes a talk with a friend can help. Sometimes you might want to enlist the help of a psychotherapist for larger, more complex, chronic, interpersonal issues. Most dietitians are not psychotherapists (though, if you're lucky enough to know both, you're in excellent hands!). However, a dietitian can help you process feelings as they relate to your food behavior—and your food parenting behavior. (In every case—friend, dietitian, or psychotherapist—just be sure you know who you're talking to. Unfortunately, I've had clients tell me from time to time that their therapist told them that losing weight would help them with the issues at hand. When it comes to charged and polarizing issues such as eating and weight, choosing friends and professionals who are anti-diet and weight neutral is your best bet; otherwise, you run the risk of creating even more internal conflict or a fracturing a friendship.)

You can also do this work on your own. Use the **Reflection** questions at the end of this chapter to help you get more clarity on what attitudes and beliefs about food might underlie your feelings and behaviors with eating. You can also use the next chapter on Nutrition to develop a clearer, more nutritional perspective on and education about nutrition, unfettered by the persuasion of those outside influences. Together, they can help you feel more open, relaxed, and accepting of your daughter's—and your own—food preferences and eating style.

ACCEPTANCE MAKES HEALTHY EATING EASIER

Bravely becoming more self-aware of your own feelings and ultimately more accepting of yourself and your daughter will have direct positive impacts on her self-esteem and her overall eating well-being. Remember those four areas of eating competence that are so crucial to being a happy, healthy eater? Having a positive, open, and accepting attitude towards a wide variety of foods helps in the following ways.

Acceptance Makes Intuitive Eating Easier. Being more accepting of food increases internal regulation, one of the four realms of eating competence. When we accept the fact that our daughter loves for instance, mac and cheese, we can allow her to eat it in an amount that is filling and satisfying to her and thus support her in eating according to her own needs. We will be able to resist the urge to limit or restrict the amount she eats, which increases her own comfort around these foods. The more we learn to lean into acceptance rather than fear, we will be able to serve more often and with less restraint or inner turmoil. This also helps her feel more relaxed and reassured that she doesn't need to hoard extra helpings because she might not get it again, or feel guilt or shame for enjoying it. We don't want her to feel that she needs to repent by limiting her food at the next meal or doubling up on a workout tomorrow.

Acceptance Makes Learning to Like New Foods Easier. When we accept our daughter's food preferences and appetite, we also support her in feeling comfortable exploring new foods. If she can trust that you won't force her to eat a food she doesn't like, she comes to the table feeling much more relaxed and confident about herself and her eating, qualities that have the added bonus of helping her feel the courage and curiosity it takes to try a new thing (like baked salmon or marinated artichokes) in the first place. Being accepting of your daughter's willingness (or unwillingness) to try new foods, as well as the pace she takes to get there, is the best way to support her in growing with food.

Finally, many of the foods that diet and health culture typically tell us are "unhealthy" aren't the nutritional demons we think they are. Checking our own attitudes about foods (which we'll do next in the chapter on Nutrition) can make it so much easier to accept our daughters' foods preferences, idiosyncrasies, and peccadilloes without judgment or worry in the first place, and that positive, nonjudgmental approach is the best way to open up the door for her to feel more confidence and less fear when it comes to trying new things on her own.

Acceptance Makes Meal Planning Easier. When we are solid in our feelings about food and have an attitude of acceptance, meal planning becomes much less fraught with problems. When we aren't afraid of our daughter eating too much starch, for example, and we don't judge a frozen dinner or regard the fact that we quickly put together a bowl of pasta and sauce as "horrible," "lazy," or "unhealthy," we can make coming to the table regularly much easier.

Back in my dieting days, there were countless times when I felt so overwhelmed by the decision of "what to eat" that I didn't end up eating anything at all. There were so many competing narratives in my head about every single option that I'd leave the work cafeteria, restaurant, or my own refrigerator with empty hands. Trying to decide with all of the conflict in my mind was impossible: One food was too high in carbohydrates or not high enough in protein; another was the right amount of protein but too much fat; another had the right type of fat but was coupled with some sugar; another was just the right nutritional balance in terms of whatever particular diet or eating regimen I was following, but I couldn't bear to eat it because of the taste; while yet another was something I knew to be filling and delicious but was too high in calories or the latest form of ingredient 'witchcraft' that I thought I'd never survive. Dieters aren't the only ones who get paralyzed by food fears; parents report that feeling burdened and concerned about making meals healthy enough for their kids is one of the reasons they avoid making family meals at all.[4] This is a perfect illustration of letting *perfect* be the enemy of the *good*.

Today, I lead with pleasure and use what Satter calls "good sense" when it comes to choosing what to eat and what to feed my girls. That means I prioritize us eating over making meals perfect. I don't just toss a bag of Sour Patch Kids on the table (although I would, if that's all we had and everyone was starving); it means I take into account what's tasty and will fill us up, and I balance out the rest of the day and make choices based on what's available. In other words, if I can't make or eat a picture-perfect, healthy meal, then I use good sense to make do with what we've got—and I do it in an accepting, non-judgmental way, so we can easily enjoy it. Being accepting of our abilities and limitations when it comes to planning, cooking, and shopping, can make eating together enjoyable, and in a positive way have it happen more often. Show yourself compassion, give yourself permission for feeding your children the best you can based on their likes and abilities, and use whatever resources you have available at any given meal.

Acceptance Improves Lifelong Eating. When we accept our daughter's food preferences, eating style, and body weight, we help her have positive attitudes about eating. With that strength, she is better able to work on the other areas of her eating competence, which, as you remember, will bolster her protection against disordered eating. She will become more confident in her own style of eating and food preferences, even if they are in contradiction to what diet culture or other influential people think.

IFM Touchstone: *Acceptance*

What is one issue with regarding to eating behavior or body that you feel you are least accepting of? What is one action you can take to help you increase acceptance? For example, *I intend to avoid putting myself down in front of my daughter* or *I intend to be clear and direct when I give my daughter an instruction about food.*

Eating is meant to be a joyful, nourishing, and self-directed experience. In order for our daughters to be physically, emotionally, and socially healthy eaters, we need them to come to the table feeling confident, comfortable, and expectant of a positive experience that *honors*—not disapproves of or dismisses—their preferences, eating abilities, and temperament. We also need to respect their individual body signals such as appetite, hunger, and fullness. Our acceptance of who they are with their eating, as well as our belief that they can grow and improve, is the best way to help them be and stay happy, healthy eaters.

REFLECTIONS FOR ACCEPTANCE

- *What were your parents' attitudes towards eating? Was pleasure in food a priority? Was eating for health a priority? Was eating the most economical or fastest meal a priority?*

- *Was eating itself a priority? In other words, were meals planned in advance—or was food grabbed on the fly? What about eating together as a family—was that a priority? Or was it each person for themselves?*

- *Was food always available to you? Or do you remember worrying about getting enough or getting enough of the foods you really enjoyed?*

- *What is your own attitude toward food now? Do you think of foods based on their nutritional value—or lack thereof? Or do you prioritize taste and pleasure? When you decided what to eat for lunch yesterday, did you choose based on nutrition content? Taste? Or convenience?*

- *What's something that was said to you as a child about food or eating that you have caught yourself saying to your daughter? What's the tone behind it? Is it shaming and criticizing or positive, open, and accepting?*

CHAPTER EIGHT
SIMPLIFYING NUTRITION

"A little simplification would be the first step
toward rational living, I think."

—*Eleanor Roosevelt*

I REMEMBER WITH CRYSTAL CLARITY THE DAY I REALIZED I needed to revamp the way I practiced nutrition forever. I walked out of the exam room where I typically saw patients, around the corner, down the hall, and through the heavy, fire-proof door that pushed into the windowless office I shared with a thoughtful, intelligent social worker. I dumped the weight of my body, heavy with everything I just heard in my last session, into my chair. Before she had a chance to speak, I swiveled to face her and exclaimed, "Everyone has gone mad!" To her wide eyes, I added, "A parent just asked me if apples are HEALTHY." If they were crossing fruit off the list of foods that are okay to eat, what would be next? That was the moment I realized I needed to reframe the way I talked to parents about nutrition—or quit working as a dietitian.

Forty-five minutes earlier, I had started a session with 10-year-old Jeremy, who was talkative, confident, and lively. It was January and he was referred to me due to a bump up in BMI percentile, a change that had occurred since the start of the school year the previous fall. As far as I could tell, Jeremy was a fairly balanced eater who enjoyed a lot of different foods, ate on a pretty regular schedule, and was fortunate enough to have parents who could afford to send him to tennis lessons as well as to Switzerland for summer camp. This beaming young man was also fortunate enough to have not just his mother, but also his maternal grandmother, take an interest in his eating and join him in the visit. Grandma seemed particularly invested in addressing Jeremy's changing BMI, sharing that "he looked so beautiful" when he came home from camp because he'd "slimmed down," and encouraging him to "confess to the junk food," as she put it. He sheepishly responded by telling me that a classmate had been stowing Oreos in his locker and sometimes he shared them.

From my perspective, the uptick in weight made sense. This child has come off a very active summer and transitioned back to living in New York City, with long, sedentary days at a private academy. He was also in a completely new school, which he took a cab to instead of walking. His lunchtime eating habits were new, too. The Oreos were not the problem. There wasn't even a question about allowing the classically maligned foods like cookies and french fries; this family was way beyond that and wanted to account for every possible offender. Mom asked, "Are apples okay? He really likes them, but aren't they too 'carby'?" They were considering turning on a food that, not too long ago, was considered the epitome of healthy eating.

I remember looking at Jeremy, a high achiever and an aim-to-pleaser who was taking notes. It took me a moment to recalibrate. *Were they really asking me if apples were okay to eat?*

A look around the room made me realize that, yes, that was exactly what all three of them were asking me! The idea that an apple a day could help keep the doctor away was officially dead. This family's question was the proverbial straw that broke this camel's back. People, including parents, are overwhelmed by a crippling amount of nutrition information, which can at times be complex and contradictory. Ironically, all that information can get in the way of being and raising a healthy eater.

After that visit, I vowed to keep nutrition as simple as possible and to ease food fears—not fan them—at every opportunity. If you've been surprised to find information on nutrition as one of the last chapters (and the last piece of the IFM) in a book about helping raise healthy eaters, you may now better understand the reason. While good nutritional health is acquired by eating a wide variety of nutritious foods, so much comes before being able to eat those foods in calm, positive, and consistent ways. Our feelings and attitudes about foods, body, and weight dictate so much of our eating behaviors—and if we are a parent, our food parenting approach—that it'd be futile to address the *whats* of eating first. Now that we've developed better insights into *how* to eat to be well—what at NourishHer we refer to as essential eating skills (EES)—we can start thinking more closely about the types of foods we eat. If you find this information overwhelms you or distracts from protecting your daughter from a dieting mentality or an ability to be flexible around food, I recommend saving it for a future time (or reaching out for support from a professional who can help you incorporate it in a positive, helpful way).

In this chapter, you will learn the essentials of good, basic nutrition for children. This includes making sure your daughter eats enough food to meet her needs for growth as well as enough variety, a hallmark of good nutritional health, since it allows for getting enough of various nutrients. I share what tends to make nutrition feel complicated, what nutrients and food groups to focus on, portion size information, tips for meal and snack planning, and finally, answers to some common questions. In the end, I hope you and your daughter will never feel the need to ask questions about whether apples or chips or the number two special at your favorite convenience food restaurant is healthy or too 'carby' before you eat it.

WHY 'SHOULD' AND 'EAT' DON'T GO TOGETHER

When you look up the word "should" in the Oxford dictionary, you find it is "used to indicate obligation, duty, or correctness, typically when criticizing someone's actions." In my mind, should is a dirty word that brings about all kinds of inner turmoil, making us feel guilt and question our actions, as well as steering us away from what's right for us.

I am against all manner of shoulds, particularly when it comes to talking about eating. That even goes for, "You should avoid all rules and just eat what you love in the amounts that feels right." There's no one right food to eat nor one right way of eating; there are only the facts of what is and then our individual decision to apply that information in the way that works best for us.

I actively avoid rigid rules and shoulds when it comes to nutrition counseling. That can frustrate clients; so many of us want to be told what and how much to eat. On the other hand, there are certain principles or facts about nutrition that I think are helpful to understand. There are certain 'basics' about macronutrients and micronutrients and how they work in the body that can help empower women to understand their own physiology, as well as that of the girls they are raising.

Developing a strong understanding of core nutrition principles can protect us and our daughters from the false promises of food manufacturers, best-selling (and often 'credential-less' or under-credentialed) authors, celebrities, social media superstars, and even medical professionals. There are an endless number of uninformed 'experts' who make false, misleading, or unsubstantiated claims about foods and eating. Those claims are most often directed at women; thus, we need to be extra equipped to arm ourselves and our daughters against them.

My goal is to avoid telling you exactly what you or your daughter should eat and instead give you the vital and helpful nutritional information you need to make informed choices that best serve you and your family. These are the basics of nutrition.

THINK LIKE A REGISTERED DIETITIAN (RD)

Before I became an RD, my attitudes towards food and my decisions about eating were dominated by diet and health culture and a fear of gaining weight and developing a disease. A cookie was a sugary, tempting treat that I felt needed to be limited to snack time or dessert, if allowed at all. A hamburger was a high calorie indulgence that might cause high blood pressure or heart disease. A leafy salad felt safe and a 'should' food while the creamy dressing offered with it did not.

After I became an RD, I saw foods in a very different light. Now there's less charge, emotion, and bias involved. I see a chocolate chip cookie, for example, as a source of carbohydrates, both simple and complex, and saturated fat, as well as some B vitamins and iron. A hamburger has iron, protein, fat, B12, and zinc. A salad is high in antioxidants and vitamins, depending on the greens used; however, it's not going to be a lot of calories nor filling unless a dressing with fat is added and, when it comes to those vitamins, a tremendous amount of lettuce would need to be eaten in order to reach a daily recommended amount.

In other words, now I think of foods in terms of what they have to offer. And while the nutrients in them don't change, their nutritional value does, relative to what each individual person needs. Those needs differ from person to person depending on a multitude of factors, including everything from age, gender, diagnosis, disease risk, accessibility, environment, to skill level in terms of eating and cooking. In other words, how healthy or unhealthy a food is, depends first and foremost on context.

In some cases, the context is clear to me—for example, a client tells me she has diabetes or I know she's about to enter puberty, or that she has an allergy to peanuts. Sometimes the context is not so clear; I might not know she has a sister who has recovered from an eating disorder, a parent who isn't home from work in time to cook dinner, that she's about to get braces, or that access to affordable food is a problem. Those are factors I'd have to dig for, and something many of the people who freely give out eating advice fail to consider.

Some simple examples of how context can change the value of foods; peanut butter is a good source of fat and protein and calories, making it a highly valuable food for a growing child, yet a teaspoon could render an entire meal deadly in the case of someone who's allergic to peanuts. A bag of popcorn labeled "skinny" could be a good, portable snack and source of fiber for one child, and a trigger food to someone who's healing from restriction or totally useless to a child who just got braces. A high-fiber, high-fat food like avocado might be good for someone managing their blood sugar who is prone to inflammation or constipation, yet those same nutrients could make it too filling for a child who is having trouble eating enough food or gaining weight. Skittles could be considered a bad idea for a younger child because of the risk of choking and their lack of vitamins and minerals, yet fifteen Skittles could save the life of a child with type 1 diabetes. A bag of Cheetos might have too much sodium for someone with high blood pressure, but be a much-needed source of calories and even some iron, potassium, and calcium for a child whose family doesn't have the time or money to provide another option for a snack.

I'm sharing this perspective with you to help open minds and simplify nutrition. Before dietitians make any nutrition-related recommendations for our clients and patients, we always do a thorough assessment first to provide context. We figure out where you are, and then work from there. This is yet another reason why diets don't work. Your individual experience, preferences, and circumstances—*your* context—gets completely negated from the conversation.

SIMPLIFYING NUTRITION

For the purpose of this book, I'm going to take only one thing for granted: that you're thinking of food with your growing daughter in mind. With that context in mind, our primary goals in this discussion are two-fold: that she gets enough *energy* (i.e., calories) consistently and enough *variety* (particularly in vitamins and minerals).

MACRONUTRIENTS

Macronutrients are larger nutrients that provide energy in the form of calories. Energy is the primary fuel for a growing body. Remember, even if your daughter has reached an age where she has finished growing in height, she is still growing. Organs such as her brain and bones continue to grow into her early twenties. As a primary concern, we want to make sure our daughter is getting enough macronutrients, which make up the bulk of her eating and fill her energy needs.

To be clear, there are three times of macronutrients: carbohydrates, protein, and fat. Carbohydrates and protein each have four calories per gram while fat has nine calories, meaning it provides a bigger energy boost per gram. Each macronutrient has a different function, which is why all three are important to include in most girls' diets. Carbohydrates can be simple or complex (many simple sugars chained together) and both are turned into glucose when eaten and used primarily for energy. Protein is considered a building block, and it is used to provide structure and repair cells including bones, muscles, and tissues. It can also be broken down to provide energy. Fat is used for energy, growth, and cell structure, particularly in the brain, to assist in the absorption of fat-soluble vitamins, to help make hormones, and for padding and protection, as well as to help keep the body warm.

Yes, different types of macronutrients function slightly differently in the body. Complex carbohydrates include varying amounts of fiber (a non-digestible form of carbohydrate) move more slowly through the gut than those that are simple. Protein is built from a combination of smaller parts called amino acids, and foods do not contain all the essential ones, rendering them incomplete (another reason why variety is key). Fats can be broken down into saturated and unsaturated, and have different secondary impacts on the body. Saturated fats come from animal foods and are linked with increased inflammation and LDL or "bad" cholesterol, while unsaturated fats come from plant foods and do the opposite, easing inflammation and improving cholesterol.

So long as your daughter isn't actively avoiding any one nutrient (such as carbohydrates or fat, for example) and you're involved in planning or helping her plan meals and snacks, ensuring your daughter gets enough macronutrients can be fairly easy. Carbohydrates are found primarily in grains, fruits, and starchy vegetables. Protein is found primarily in fish, meats, poultry, eggs, and dairy. Fat is found primarily in oils, nuts, some fish, and some animal foods, such as full fat dairy. Most foods have more than one macronutrient and, in some cases, all three.

If your daughter does have a particular health condition or concern that's diet-related (such as high cholesterol, diabetes, or insulin resistance), consult a pediatric dietitian to get recommendations and a more nuanced understanding of it and how different types each of these three macronutrients impact her condition. Otherwise, I'd focus on improving her overall eating skills and competence as she grows by helping her learn to enjoy a variety of foods without stress so as to take in all three macronutrients.

MICRONUTRIENTS

Micronutrients are much less important calorically; however, they are absolutely crucial to an endless list of bodily functions, including creating energy and growth.

Micronutrients include vitamins, minerals, and phytochemicals such as flavonoids, flavones, catechins, polyphenols, and phytoestrogens. Micronutrients are vital to just about everything our body does, including blood pressure regulation, muscle contractions, immunity, nervous system growth and activity, inflammation reduction, cancer prevention, cognition, enzyme production, metabolism, and a whole host of other functions.

There are at least 30 micronutrients that our body cannot make, and none of them are found in any one food, which is why helping our daughter with variety is more important to her overall nutritional health than teaching her to have limits. When our daughters start limiting foods, such as with dieting and restrictive styles of healthy eating, they put themselves at risk of getting insufficient micronutrients that their body needs. And, unlike limiting calories, the risks might not be visually obvious. A body deprived of vitamin B12, which can occur on a vegan diet, can cause unclear symptoms, such as confusion, depression, and memory issues.

Micronutrients are in many foods; however, fruits and vegetables tend to contain the highest amounts of vitamins, minerals, and phytochemicals per gram or ounce. For that reason, I recommend offering at least one fruit or vegetable (or food that contains a fruit or vegetable) with every meal or snack as often as you can, as well as enjoying them alongside her. As we learned earlier, there's no need to pressure or prompt her to eat it. Making it pleasant and enjoyable, including in preparation style (yes, butter on vegetables or something sweet on bitter is okay so long as it improves taste and makes it more appealing to eat).

When it comes to micronutrients, many parents ask me if they can give their daughter a supplement. Yes, you can (although I recommend you do so with the guidance of your pediatrician or dietitian). Vitamin D, in particular, can be difficult to get in sufficient amounts from food alone. Typically, the body would rely on sunlight to make the vitamin. If you live in certain areas such as Northeastern United States, or routinely wear sunscreen when outdoors, then sufficient exposure can be limited and vitamin D levels decline. Calcium, too, can be considered if your daughter is vegan or eats less than two to three servings of dairy foods daily. If you think your daughter might need a supplement, speak to your pediatrician or registered dietitian for advice on the amounts and best ways to take it.

Even if you do decide to supplement, it's best to get nutrients from food sources whenever possible. Many nutrients such as vitamins and minerals work synergistically with one another; for example, some vitamins such as A, D, E, and K can only be absorbed in the presence of fat. Also, many lesser-known phytochemicals found in fruits and vegetables aren't available in supplements. You can rely on a supplement as a fail-safe while you're working towards better eating or when eating a variety of micronutrient-containing foods is not possible.

Despite these facts, I have found that for the majority of healthy children, figuring out the nuances of each micronutrient can be overwhelming and confusing. I've pulled out a few nutrients to be extra aware of for girls, as these are the specific ones they either tend to be low in or need extra amounts of (see chart on page 191). However, unless it's absolutely necessary due to a food-related diagnosis, I avoid going much deeper into nutrition. Having too much information when making decisions about what to eat and how to prepare it causes both parents and children to start stressing about eating and feeding, limiting food groups, and using less appetizing preparation styles. All this takes away from the most important nutritional task at hand—making sure your child is getting enough energy and enough variety in their foods.

GIRL-SPECIFIC NUTRITION

Growing up, every time I complained about feeling tired, my mother's response would be, "Well, you don't eat enough protein." If it seems like an antiquated concern, I've found that, aside from sugar (which we will get to in a moment), not getting enough protein is still an alive-and-well-worry I hear from the majority of mothers I work with. The good news is that protein probably isn't a nutrient you need to be watching out for when it comes to our daughters' diets. It's estimated that the majority of kids in the United States don't just meet but exceed the recommended amounts, which is something that I have found to be true even among girls I've worked with who've had very limited food intake.

What nutrients might we be more focused on to worry about? In general, the nutrients I pay closest attention to when screening the diets of school age, adolescent, and teen girls include adequate overall macronutrients for energy needs (there's currently a tendency to limit carbohydrates, in particular, thanks to the popularity of certain weight loss diets), as well as iron, calcium, vitamin D, magnesium, and fiber. More details on the reasons I hit on those five as well as which foods contain them can be found in the chart below. (When girls have limited variety due to restricting certain foods or food groups the list grows slightly longer than what is included here, and the consequences can be more significant in a growing child than in an adult, which is one of the reasons why I recommend focusing on increasing variety and avoid, fearing, and eliminating foods without a medical reason.)

GIRL-SPECIFIC NUTRIENTS

	IRON	CALCIUM	VITAMIN D	MAGNESIUM	FIBER
Why Girls	While boys tend to meet their iron needs, girls fall short due to losses from menstruation, putting them at risk for iron deficiency. Dieting (skipping meals, cutting out food groups) will also put them at risk for not meeting the recommended amounts.	Peak bone accumulation happens in girls between ages 11 and 14. Girls in this age meet only about 60 percent of their needs. This is thought to be due to fears among girls that calcium-containing foods cause weight gain.	Girls are less likely to have adequate D levels than boys, with only 50 percent meeting recommended intakes and rates being even lower when sorted by ethnicity. African American and Mexican American girls are more at risk possibly due to less D being absorbed by darker skin tones.	A whopping 89 percent of girls ages 14 to 18 don't get enough magnesium in their diets. Avoiding a magnesium shortfall may help girls get better sleep, have more balanced moods, and have better concentration, in addition to preventing bone loss as they age.	Since girls are more prone to restriction, they may not be getting enough fiber and, conversely, since it is known to suppress appetite, they may also overeat fiber, which can cause secondary problems such as bloating and cramping, as well as crowding out room in the diet for other micronutrient containing foods. With this nutrient, it's important to make sure girls are getting enough and not too much.
Where to Find It	Animal foods such as beef, turkey, and chicken contain a highly absorbable form of iron called heme. Iron-fortified cereals, lentils, spinach, oatmeal, and bread made with fortified flour also contain iron though in a less well-absorbed form (nonheme).	Dairy foods such as cow's milk (as well as calcium-fortified milk alternatives), cheese, ice cream and yogurt. Calcium-fortified orange juice and cereals. Some vegetables such as broccoli and spinach, though multiple servings are needed to meet needs.	Salmon, vitamin-D-fortified orange juice, full, low, and nonfat milk (including some milk alternatives such as almond, oat, rice, and soy), and vitamin D supplements.	Almonds, cashews, peanut butter, seeds, yogurt, and leafy greens.	Nuts, seeds, fruits, vegetables, beans, and whole grains such as oats, brown rice, and popcorn, as well as breads and flours made from whole grains

To make sure your daughter is getting enough of the vitamins and minerals above, you can offer her the whole foods listed above as well as packaged foods that include those foods as ingredients. When unsure, iron, calcium, and vitamin D are listed at the bottom of the nutrition facts label. When choosing between foods or brands, opt for foods that contain the highest percentages when possible.

Nutrition Facts

8 servings per container

Serving size   2/3 cup (55g)

Amount per serving

Calories   230

	% Daily Value*
Total Fat 8g	**10%**
Saturated Fat 1g	**5%**
Trans Fat 0g	
Cholesterol 0mg	**0%**
Sodium 160mg	**7%**
Total Carbohydrate 37g	**13%**
Dietary Fiber 4g	**14%**
Total Su...	
...ncludes 10g Added Sugars	**20%**
Prot...	
Vitamin D 2mcg	10%
Calcium 260mg	20%
Iron 8mg	45%
Potassium 240mg	6%

...% Daily Value (DV) tells you how much... ...a day is used for general nutrition advice.

HUNGER AND FULLNESS

If you start thinking like an RD, then you'll also be able to see foods in terms of how satisfying they may or may not be. Foods may be satisfying based on both their macronutrient content (which is more objective) and how appetizing they may be (which is more subjective and differs from person to person). Understanding both aspects of fullness is important and can help you make sure you daughter is a happy, well-nourished eater.

Hunger can be used to describe how empty your body feels in a physical sense. A gurgling belly, feeling irritable or lightheaded, or being extremely focused on foods can all be signs of physical hunger. Different macronutrients have different impacts on how physically full we feel after eating, which is why including all three is an important part of good nutrition.

Carbohydrates—particularly those that are low in fiber—can make you feel full almost immediately after eating them, as they digest quickly. They give us a quick satiety. Simple carbs—such as those that are low in fiber and high in sugar—act quickly on satisfaction, while more complex ones have a slight delay. Fat and protein take longer to digest; therefore, the energy is released into your system on a longer delay, yet the feeling of fullness can last longer. An illustration of this phenomenon follows.

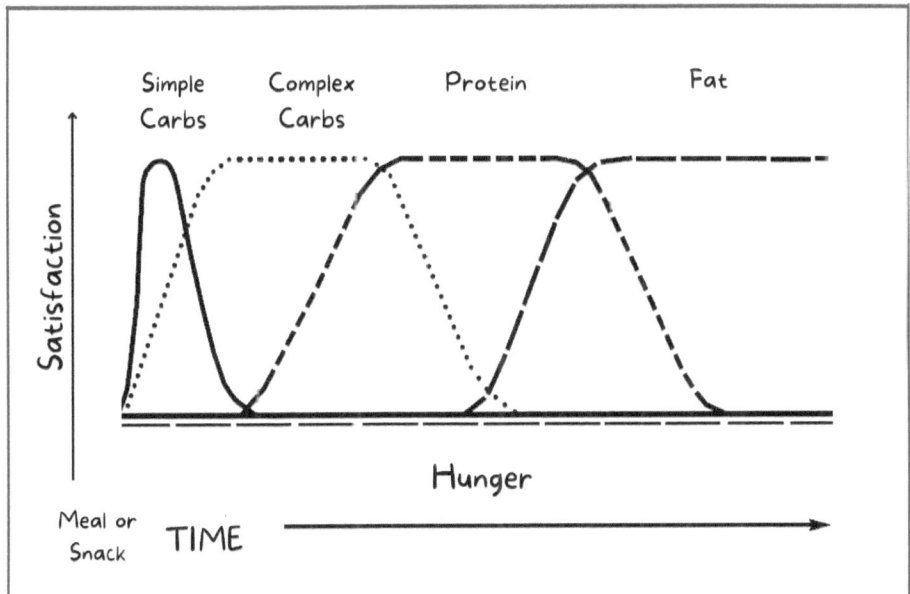

Adapted from Figure G.5 "Satiety from Consuming Sugar, Starch, Protein, and Fat" in Ellyn Satter's *Secrets of Feeding a Health Family* Appendix G "Foods that help regulation."

Copyright © Ellyn Satter. Reproduced with permission from *Secrets of Feeding a Healthy Family: How to Eat, How to Raise Good Eaters, How to Cook.* For more information, go to www.EllynSatterInstitute.org.

When we think about eliminating a macronutrient, we can start to understand how we will shortchange not only our daughter's nutrient intake, but also the satisfaction of any given food or meal. To help us feel satisfied initially and have that feeling last for an extended time (until the next scheduled meal or snack time), it's helpful to include a blend of carbohydrates, protein, and fats.

A snack without any carbohydrates—like a cheese stick— might not be satisfying to your daughter, since it lacks that initial burst of fullness. Likewise, a snack of only carbohydrates—no matter how much—such as a large bag of Pirate's Booty might be initially satisfying, but leave her feeling hungry and looking for more food a short while later. Also, when hunger is very high, those foods that satisfy us quickly—such as sugary carbohydrates—become even more appealing, since our body knows we can get what we need much faster from them.

Since physical fullness is more objective, we can somewhat account for the specific sensation by learning more about how macronutrients work in the body and making sure we use them to our advantage when eating and offering them to our kids. If you're trying to help your daughter feel fuller longer, then include macronutrients that have longer staying power, such as proteins and fats (as evidenced by the longer horizontal lines in the illustration above). If you're trying to help your daughter increase her food intake, include foods with shorter staying power (such as simple carbohydrates) to help make sure she's interested in eating again at the next meal.

Appetite. In addition to satisfying hunger, we also want to satisfy our appetite. Appetite refers to how enjoyable a food is, which is more sub-jective and can change from person to person throughout life. Foods that your daughter finds appetizing are only known to her and can change over time as her experience and exposures grow.

I'M STUFFED & STILL HUNGRY

To really feel satisfied, foods need to appeal to *both* our physical hunger and our appetite. Since they are based on different things—physical fullness or pleasure—these two different measures of satisfaction have different stopping points. This explains why sometimes we may feel physically full—stuffed, even—and still have an urge or desire to eat more.

If we choose only foods that are physically filling, such as a piece of grilled chicken, we can be left still wanting to eat other more appetizing foods, such as the slice of cheesy, delicious-smelling pizza on the plate of the person sitting next to us. It also explains how a slice of chocolate cake can seem appealing even after a filling dinner. When you understand the importance of satisfying appetite, it can make it easier to see the importance of including highly enjoyable foods in meals and snacks.

If your daughter is eating a large amount of filling nutrients, but still says she's hungry, you might try appealing to her appetite—or enjoyment of foods—instead. I actually find that overlooking the appetizing impact of foods is one reason many of my clients overeat on diets. To solve this problem, create meals that include both filling and enjoyable food combinations that help hit the fullness and satisfying feelings at the same time.

We also need to teach our daughters to notice the sensations of satisfaction. When our hunger is satisfied, we start to notice our body feeling physically full. When our appetite is satisfied, we start to notice that food begins to not taste as good. Of course, we need to be relaxed and paying close attention to our body's sensations to notice either. This is another benefit to helping yourself and your daughter keep calm and cool at meals as opposed to feeling stressed and tense.

ALL FOODS HAVE NUTRITION

In the previous chapter, I talked a lot about how our attitudes about foods can make eating an emotional experience filled with confusion, fear, guilt, and shame. If that wasn't reason enough to avoid labeling foods as good and bad, healthy and unhealthy, super and junk, here's what might be an even better reason—nutritionally speaking, those labels aren't true.

All foods have nutritional value and are nourishing. Humans are designed to thrive while eating a variety of foods in a variety of different ways. Plus, as mentioned earlier, the nutritional value of food changes significantly based on context; a food that might work well for your body and situation might not work for someone else. Even when we know which nutrients are broadly needed, the sources they might come from and ways they are prepared and combinations that they are eaten with are extremely complex. As you might have noticed in reading about nutrients above, most foods cross the divide and contain multiple macronutrients and micronutrients. Lentils contain protein, carbohydrates, and iron. Ice cream contains simple carbohydrates as well as protein, calcium, and vitamin D. A chicken tender (which parents always apologize for letting their kids eat) contains protein, carbs, and fat, plus a good source of vitamin B6, niacin, selenium, and phosphorus. Avocado includes fat, fiber, and vitamin C. Guacamole has all of that, plus extra vitamin C and phytochemicals from the tomatoes, onion, and garlic. Chips and guac contain all those nutrients, plus some complex carbohydrates (including fiber) and a bit of protein.

Of course, certain foods contain different nutrients in different amounts, including some that, in some contexts, we might want to limit (saturated fat and sodium, for example, for those at risk for heart disease.) However, that doesn't negate all the other nutrition that's available within that food. In the case of a growing body with high nutrient needs, it's best to focus on what's nutritious and delicious in a food over what's to fear. Having an open mind can prevent your daughter from cutting out foods and ultimately give her the best chance of getting the variety of nutrients she needs for optimal health, well-being, and growth.

To help our daughters get enough food and enough variety, I recommend opting for a policy of *food neutrality*. If you can do your best to see what needed nutrients foods *do* have—as opposed to what they lack, and think about the positive function of those nutrients—you'll feel less stressed and be able to raise a daughter who's getting all the nutrition she needs.

MEAL-PLANNING TIPS

When it comes to meal planning, keep these tips in mind and you'll keep stress low while also ensuring your daughter eats well and receives the right nutrition.

A rule-of-thumb I recommend is to aim to offer all three macro-nutrients at meals and two of the three at snacks. For example, rice (carbohydrate) plus chicken (protein) plus oil (fat) on vegetables. Or eggs (protein), plus butter (fat), plus toast (carbohydrate). Or for a snack, Greek yogurt (protein) plus berries (carbohydrate) or a cheese stick (protein) plus crackers (carbohydrate) or Oreos (carbohydrate) plus almonds (protein).

For every meal or snack, do your best to include one source of fruit or vegetable as a way to increase micronutrient content. (Fruits and starchy vegetables such as potatoes, corn, or peas might double as the carbohydrate source.) I recommend thinking of fruits and vegetables interchangeably, since they both are excellent sources of micronutrients. Both cantaloupe and cauliflower contain potassium, for example. Both kiwi and broccoli are good sources of vitamin C. Since color indicates the availability of different nutrients, opt for increasing variety in color across both fruits and vegetables, as opposed to pushing vegetables over fruits.

Try your best to offer a variety of foods over the course of the day and even through the week. Give yourself some leeway and think about how you can balance eating from day to day with a variety of foods, as opposed to perfecting every meal.

Remember from the chapter on trust: For best results with our daughters' eating, our job as parents and feeders is to plan balanced meals and offer foods. Our daughters' job is to decide if and how much to eat.

WHAT ABOUT SUGAR?

I know what you're thinking: But what about sugar? I thought of pulling sugar out and giving it its own chapter, since it is the thing that tends to cause the most conflict, guilt, and confusion between parents and kids. Then I thought, heck no! Why play into that mentality? Let me keep it short and sweet instead (pun intended).

You may have heard claims that sugar is as addictive, harmful, and toxic as drugs such as alcohol and cocaine. While any google search can turn up studies that show sugar is neurochemically rewarding, the evidence that it causes the same addictive behaviors or toxic side effects is not strong. For one, rats in these studies are fed sugar irregularly or in near-starving states (not similar to real life unless you're severely restricting and then offered only sugar). Second, the boost of dopamine (a brain chemical involved in pleasure, reward, and motivation) rats get from sugar wears off after repeated exposure, which is not what happens with drugs such as cocaine. As far as I am aware, there's no significant studies done in humans that sugar is toxic or addictive.

With this in mind, there's no reason that an otherwise healthy person needs to severely limit, restrict, or have a strong set of rules around it. If you have trouble believing me, I don't blame you. The demonizing of sugar is a true and real thing, particularly by proponents of diet culture. The scientific truth is: Sugar is pleasurable and neurochemically rewarding. Unlike drugs, it has significant nutritional value—and the fact that we enjoy (or even crave) it may be an evolutionary function, ensuring we seek it out and eat it! Scientifically speaking, once digested and absorbed, sugar (aka glucose) from candy or cake has the same as nutritional value as sugar (also glucose) you get from any other carbohydrate source, such as whole grains (like oatmeal), vegetables (like potatoes), and legumes (like chickpeas and lentils).

If you truly can't get over your fear of sugar and loosen the reins when eating it, if you really want to hold tight to the idea that sugar is not something you can trust her around and is a threat to her health, I ask you to consider this: How will the rules you have around sugar help her in the long run? How will the restrictions impact her ability to enjoy sugary foods in a neutral way, once you no longer can enforce the rules or limits? Do the rules you have in place seem to be helping her enjoy sugary foods in calm and balanced ways when she is on her own?

Speaking from personal experience as someone with a sweet tooth, as once a young girl who was told when she enjoyed sweets and treats "You'll be sorry one day," and as a professional who has studied both the nutritional and behavioral science, I don't recommend instituting tight control around sugary foods. Instead, I encourage you to incorporate them into your weekly menus as you would other carbohydrates and do your best to keep a neutral attitude about how much or how little your child decides to eat or seems to enjoy. With this approach, they stand the best shot of regarding these foods the same way when they're presented with them at parties, supermarkets, vending machines, grandma's house, or other places.

"My Daughter Needs a Special Diet." Many of us are lucky in the sense that the majority of kids can eat a wide variety of foods to be healthy. Eating regularly and reliably are the only bits we need to focus on to raise a healthy eater. However, many of us—myself included—also have special diseases or disorders that require paying close attention to foods, nutritional content, additives, and composition. If your child has type 1 diabetes, for example, counting carbohydrates is a mainstay of your day. If your child has celiac disease, vigilantly reading labels and restricting certain foods is a part of protecting her health. And if your child has a metabolic disorder such as phenylketonuria (PKU) or a food allergy, you may also have to do the same.

I won't minimize the experience of having food-related diseases or diagnoses. As a person with celiac disease, I can attest that nutrition is a little more complicated—and the added attention I need to pay to foods and my eating does cause emotional and social stress. There's a difference between paying attention to my eating due to an autoimmune condition or allergy versus paying attention to maintain a specific weight. In the first two cases, an error can be life-threatening or have serious health consequences. In the second case, the act of limiting or restricting has ambiguous, if any, health benefits. In fact, it's the act of limiting and restricting that is linked with BMI variance (or weight yo-yoing) that can have detrimental effects on our health.[1]

If your daughter does have a medical condition that requires her to pay extra special attention to her diet, figuring out that sweet spot between following the recommended restrictions on the diet—enough to keep their physical health optimized without causing their emotional and social health to tank—can be tricky. The answer will come from what you can tolerate and accept as a parent, your child's personality, and the risks to her condition. I'll give you a few examples: Type one diabetes requires close monitoring of carb intake. For some parents, having strict rules about avoiding those that raise blood sugar rather dramatically (like a heavily frosted cupcake) is not a problem. A child can take that in stride and make do with attending a party and toting along their own low-carb alternative, or saying "no thanks" to the cupcake completely. For them, restricting the sugar isn't causing major emotional stress or limiting their social life. For another child, being told they can't have the cupcake can feel stressful and isolating, even stigmatizing. Parents might choose to avoid the party altogether because of the stress it can cause, which can trip up another sort of social and emotional stress of its own. Or, those parents might value that the child be normalized in every way and decide to allow that child to enjoy the cupcake despite the blood sugar spike. To help their child suffer less emotionally and socially, they might choose to allow the sugar high and treat it with an appropriate amount of insulin—even if it takes some extra work on their part to bring it down.

In my own case of celiac disease, as a dietitian I'd recommend avoiding all gluten-containing foods, all packaged foods that say "made in a facility that also processes wheat," having gluten-containing foods in your kitchen, and even eating in gluten-containing restaurants (due to cross contamination as well as potential misunderstandings with waitstaff and food preparers). That is the official advice and what, as a professional, I consider necessary to protect a person with celiac from gluten exposure. For me personally, however, I found that while following these rules 100 percent of the time was protecting my body physically it was simultaneously causing me incredible emotional and social stress. While I never eat gluten-containing food deliberately, I do put myself at risk by eating in restaurants that serve dishes containing gluten. In reality, declining every single opportunity with family and friends to eat outside of my home was too much of an emotional burden for me to bare. For me, the stress of vigilantly avoiding every morsel of food that might contaminated was outweighing the benefit of strict protection against gluten.

These are fine lines and personal decisions that we each need to make for ourselves and our children. My point is that not all advice fits everyone. Consider your and your daughter's eating well-being.

IFM Touchstone: *Simple Nutrition*

What is one eating or food rule that may not be serving you or your daughter? What is one simple action you can take to help ease nutrition worries or make meal planning less stressful? For example, *I intend to think of all the beneficial nutrients that are in a food instead of worrying about what is missing, I intend to consider enjoyment in addition to nutrients when planning a meal or snack,* or *I intend to focus on helping my daughter feel full with more protein, fat, and fiber, instead of worrying about calories.*

REST ASSURED, YOUR DAUGHTER IS EATING WELL

If you've got the time, energy, and peace of mind to read this book, there's a good chance you've already got everything you need to keep your daughter well-nourished. If you have access to a variety of foods and the resources to buy them, if you're able to provide food regularly and reliably to yourself and your family, then rest assured you and your children have a lot of great things going on when it comes to eating and feeding. I simply can't emphasize that fact enough. Your daughter is likely well-fed.

Yes, perhaps your daughter, like the majority of girls living and eating in America, could use a little more calcium, potassium, or vitamin D and maybe she could reach for a serving of veggies more often or cut back on the candy a bit. However, all those details are inconsequential in comparison to the fact that she is regularly fed and has ample and consistent opportunities to eat a variety of safe, nutritious food.

Aside from breathing and drinking water, eating is the most important thing you will ever do.

Notice, that's all there is to it. It isn't that eating X, Y, and Z in one, two, or three amounts is the most important thing. It is simply, *eating*. Eating enough consistently is the most important and basic thing you can do to care for yourself from day to day. And when you're a parent, making sure your daughter does the same—and learns how to do it for herself—is one of the most basic and fundamental parts of taking care of her. Just do this, and you can pat yourself on the back. You don't need to quantify or qualify it by putting judgment or restrictions on food. Step one is to eat.

Simply eating is more important than checking your email or getting that call into your boss or employee or the bank or checking that your daughter's permission slip is signed or putting on the antiwrinkle cream or making sure you buy the bread with the lowest possible added sugar count. Feeding yourself—and if you're a parent, feeding your child—is it. And truth be told, any food—*any* source of energy—will do.

REFLECTIONS ON NUTRITION

- *What is your biggest concern with regard to your daughter's nutritional health? (Self-regulation, not getting enough of a specific nutrient, not eating enough variety, and eating too many packaged foods are some examples.)*

- *What is one action you can take to address this concern? How can you help her?*

- *What rule or rules do you have about food for her? For yourself? For your other children (if applicable.) Do they differ?*

- *What is the benefit of the rule(s) for your daughter's eating well-being?*

- *What, if any, might be the harm on her eating well-being?*

- *What might be a better approach for helping your daughter have a happier, healthier relationship with food?*

CHAPTER NINE
MOVEMENT

"Movement is a medicine for creating change in a person's physical, emotional, and mental states."

—*Carol Welch, Biosomatics, Movement Education, and Your Well-being*

ON OUR SECOND VISIT, MIRABEL'S MOTHER EXPLAINED THAT recently her 12-year-old had been giving her parents a lot of grief when it came to participating in swim practice. According to her mother, Mirabel had a natural athletic ability and had been a star of her swim team for as long as she could remember. Unfortunately, she was now regularly skipping practice and was no longer the energetic, happy, and talkative girl they remembered. Instead, she was sullen, moody, and angry about being made to participate at all. What had once been a point of connection between her and her mom, who had also been a competitive swimmer, had now become a point of contention.

Initially, when mom asked me to talk to her daughter about the benefits of swimming, I agreed. Physical activity, after all, is one of the first things I recommended to clients (and rely on myself!) as a way to improve many aspects of well-being, including building confidence, boosting mood, and easing stress. Yet, with mom and daughter in front of me, I realized I had made a grave mistake. The more mom spoke about how much better off Mirabel would be if she'd recommit to swimming, the more withdrawn this young girl became. When I asked her if she knew why her parents and I were concerned about her skipping swimming, her answer made everything else make sense. "Yes," she said. "It's because you guys want me to lose weight."

If you remember Mirabel from an earlier chapter, you'll also remember how concerned her parents were about her weight gain. Apparently, when she complained about wanting to have a flat belly like the ones her peers were showing off on social media, her parents jumped on it as a motivator to help her start working out more—and her love of swimming was their target of choice.

UNDERSTANDING WORKOUT CULTURE

Physical movement can be emotionally, spiritually, and physically nourishing. It's not just a practical part of existence; for some, it's essential to our entire well-being.

Regular physical activity changes our brain, improves and stabilizes our mood, which helps to avoid, ease, or eliminate depression, anxiety, and stress.[1] It also helps us to fall asleep faster and sleep deeper, meaning we wake up feeling more energized and well-rested.[2] Being active improves digestion, which relieves tummy troubles such as bloating and constipation.[3] It increases blood flow and circulation, which can help ease physical pain.[4] It wards off any number of diseases by reducing blood sugar and high blood pressure, which strengthens the heart, and bolsters the immune system.[5] Physical activity maximizes our concentration, focus, and memory.[6] It sharpens our thinking, which makes us more efficient and productive.[7] Regular activity bolsters confidence and self-esteem.[8] It makes us more aware of our body sensations, which helps us tune into our hunger and fullness.[9] Physical activity is even more powerful when done alongside others; it strengthens social ties, which helps us feel more bonded and connected with loved ones and even strangers.[10]

With all of these incredible gifts to bestow, why is it that Mirabel associates physical activity with this one thing: weight? How did her love of swimming threaten to ensnare her in the dieting trap?

Much like diet culture makes it difficult to enjoy food without developing a side dish of worry and neurosis, workout culture threatens our ability to approach movement with happiness, ease, and a delightful sort of innocence. Instead, we are mired in the idea of working out as a way to cure indiscretions committed around food or to fix perceived problems with our body's shape, size, or weight. We talk about working out and exercise as a type of drudgery that we're obligated to do in order to be good, healthy, or virtuous.

I'm not surprised when parents like Mirabel's come to me during nutrition therapy, concerned about their child's weight, and say things like, "She needs to work out! I have a treadmill and she just won't use it!" I know they, like so many of us, have been mired in the idea of working out as a way to cure (perceived) eating indiscretions and control body weight. However, I wince when I hear this; I have to resist the impulse to cover nearby children's ears. The comments feel like curse words, slicing into movement's innocence. Not only are they openly disapproving of their child's body and weight, they're also making activity feel like a type of homework they need to do to "fix" it. Worse? Their words likely will have a negative impact on their child's relationship with physical activity. When parents are critical of their child's weight, those children tend to be less active, not more. They spend less of their leisure time moving around and have lower levels of enjoyment in sports if and when they do participate.[11] If we allow it to, our profound focus on the aesthetic and health benefits of physical activity can rob us of the joy, playfulness, and innate desire to move—and threatens to do the same to our children.

And that is what I believe happened to Mirabel. While swimming used to be a source of pride, self-confidence, and pleasure, as well as a shared passion between her and her mother, once this young girl started gaining weight, everything changed. When her parents started talking about swimming as a way to burn calories, the joy of it was corrupt with rules (regarding how frequently and long she'd need to be in the pool for it to count, for example) and polluted by opportunistic benefits (such as how much more toned she'd look). Seeing swimming as a way to fix her body now overshadowed everything else the sport had meant to her.

Worse, when she began to rebel against that idea, she inadvertently also lost a significant source of self-esteem and body confidence. Without swimming, her sense of self was evaporating, while her level of stress was increasing—two changes that made it much harder to navigate the emotional chaos that was being stirred up by her changing body.

Touting weight management as a benefit of being active doesn't only steal joy from our girls. When we talk about the toning, tightening, and shrinking effects of walking, jogging, climbing, swimming, dancing, tumbling, or playing any number of other sports, we unconsciously reinforce the idea that a slimmer body is a better, more valuable body.

Additionally, by talking about the better-looking body or weight-lowering benefits of working out, we teach our daughters to search for visual evidence in the mirror or on the scale as proof that the activity is working for them. When they don't find it, they tend to lose interest, give up, or believe it isn't worth it. Young girls are especially prone to this kind of disappointment since their expectations for body perfection are so extreme to begin with.

Finally, by emphasizing the aesthetic benefits of exercise, we minimize, overlook, or fail to educate our daughters completely on the many other more significant and longer-lasting benefits we get from movement. When a young girl who knows that a long walk or fast-paced spin on her bike is a fun and effective way to feel better about a bad grade or earth-shattering fight with a best friend, she's got an easy-to-access tool that can make life's inevitable frustrations and setbacks feel more manageable. And girls who know there are many other invisible yet significant and wholly tangible benefits to moving are more likely to seek out and engage in those activities—and continue to rely on them as she gets older—compared to girls who do not.

BEING "THAT" MOM

After a Zoom call with her friends during COVID, my eight-year-old daughter came to me and said, "Mom. My friends want to start a 'workout club' with me."

"A what?" I questioned, in disbelief. "What did you say? A workout club?" My heart jumped into racing speed; my startled skin started tingling. "What on earth would that be for?" I was all kinds of fired up before she even inhaled a breath to answer.

"I don't know," she replied meekly, trying to back away from whatever it was she'd just stepped into.

"Well. You must know." I stood, dubious, waiting in deep concern.

"I don't know. Working out, I guess?" her voice trailed. As I looked into her eyes, I realized she did, in fact, have no idea what they would do. Perhaps her initial enthusiasm was less about working out and more about being flattered to be included.

"Well, I don't think that working out sounds fun," I tried to take the upper hand by redirecting the idea. "Why not rename the group? I know you've been practicing your cartwheels. What about a 'tumbling club'? Or a 'dance party club'?"

"I guess," she agreed, frightened by whatever it was that she'd just unboxed in me.

Moments later, I found myself texting the other mothers to question what was going on. Each assured me in their own way that their daughter had no concept of burning calories or working out to correct any of the other issues I thought their wanting to start working out might insinuate. "The girls want to work out to be healthy," was the gist of what they each shared with me.

While I wasn't convinced, I decided to let it go in my own way. I realized the idea for the club would likely fizzle out before it became a reality. I continued to talk about it with my daughter, suggesting that a club that focused on all of the things she likes to do movement-wise would be a lot cooler, and she earnestly agreed.

As the days went on, the workout club did fizzle for the girls. My emotions about it, however, did not. I was in constant conversation with myself, both embarrassed and defensive of my reaction. In my mind, I rehearsed conversations I might have with those mothers if the topic of our girls working out came up again. I'd explain how the idea of our little girls working out to be healthy didn't sit well with me. I'd detail my reasoning, cite research on disordered relationships with body image, and talk about the importance of reframing physical activity as an opportunity for pleasure, fun, play, and connection. I'd convince myself that I sounded helpful and rational, opposed to hypersensitive and ridiculous or absurd. I'd reassure myself that this is my area of expertise—I'm a professional—and that it made perfect sense. And yet, I worried.

As my daughter approached adolescence and teenage-hood, her sphere of influencers was growing and I had to build up my guard against this newest wave of diet-y, body-focused sway. The situation also forced me to confront the notion that, while talking to parents as a professional about dieting and disordered eating was straightforward, doing the same in my real life is much harder. Also, it felt as if more was at stake, including both my relationship with these women as well as my daughter's relationships with theirs. It made me more vulnerable and less sure that calling out the nuances in the language we were using was worth it. I questioned myself—was I being extreme?

Definitely, the answer is yes. And definitely, calling out the nuances in language about workout culture can feel uncomfortable. Yet, preserving physical activity and movement as a source of joy, play, and fun, or a source of healing, strength, solace, and power for my daughters feels well worth it. Telling girls that it's time to play, run, dance, jump, climb, compete, walk, or move as opposed to exercise or workout feels like the difference between being free of—or absorbing—all the body-sculpting, muscle-toning, and calorie-blasting connotations that go with it. And so, definitely, yes; to give my girls that freedom, I'm willing to be "that" mom.

REFRAMING THE FOCUS

It's important to avoid the cultural ideal of exercise as a moral obligation, a must-do, a punishment for our eating indiscretions, or a device we can use to craft our physical bodies to fit into cultural ideals. To support our daughters, we need to be careful of those narratives and give them plenty of opportunities to understand physical activity in a different way. Ideally, our girls will embrace the idea of regular movement as a privilege and a route to reconnect with their bodies, independent of what shape, form, intensity, or time that it takes. For some, movement may be energetic and joyful while others may regard it as simply restorative or therapeutic. No child, however, benefits by thinking of movement as mandatory, or a body re-shaper or weight-eraser.

So how do we encourage our girls to get moving without tripping up on all the negative associations, workouts, and exercises? Here are some strategies that can help, regardless of whether your daughter is naturally active or more sedentary or where she falls on the weight spectrum.

Be Mindful of Language. Referring to activity as exercising and working out can have such positive tones that the majority of us can't imagine how they might ever be harmful. And yet, for those like myself who have a history of over-reliance on exercise for calorie burning, weight control, and body toning, just the thought of someone suggesting my daughter might want to start working out sounds offensive. From my experience, young girls tend to think of working out and exercising as a means of sculpting, toning, or atoning for sins committed with food—not as a way to relax, have fun, or as a means for self-care. Instead of using the words "working out" or "exercise," which tend to sound negative, punitive, and obligatory, I recommend simple switching to words such as "movement" or "physical activity" instead. Since the words are more neutral—even fun-sounding—the response I get from those I work with when I use these words tends to be much more accepting and curious.

If your daughter herself talks about doing exercise or working out, ask her what a good workout means to her. If she answers that "it keeps you healthy" then take it a step further and ask her what being healthy means. You might be surprised that she associates the word with being thinner or burning calories, in which case it's a perfect opportunity to discuss the multiple other benefits and try to reframe her attitude towards it, perhaps as a way to emphasize the strengthening or destressing aspects instead.

Be Clear on Your Own Motives. If you're active yourself, be vocal about the non-weight-related reasons you make movement a priority so your daughter doesn't make her own assumptions. For example, share that you're running or walking regularly because it helps you clear your mind so you can solve a tough problem or increase your creativity, to help you sleep better at night, deal with stress, or it's simply that it's a gift to yourself as a daily time out. This will stop her from assuming that you're doing it to stay slim, which can inadvertently send her the message that you believe she should be doing the same thing.

Reject Misguided Marketing. If she's old enough to read, be mindful of classes you sign her up for or the activewear or equipment you buy. Whenever possible, avoid activities that openly promise to burn calories or blast body fat, as well as clothing such as butt-lifting leggings and tummy-tightening tank tops. Clothing that makes those promises are particularly tempting (since we've been so trained to believe we need these things); however, they reinforce objectifying her body by focusing on how she looks over how she feels or the clothing's actual performance. Instead, we can teach her to think more holistically about her clothing: Does it move with her? Is it comfortable? Is it warm or cooling? Will it last?

Be Open-Minded. Thanks to workout culture, many of us tend to associate physical activity with grueling things such as climbing a Stairmaster, riding a stationary bike, or taking an aerobics, boot camp, or step class. Being open to all forms, times, and types of activities, be it running around on a playground or dancing in concert with a K-Pop video, can make the opportunities for movement exponential—and they count just as much as gym workout types of exercise. Plus, enjoyment is key when it comes to helping her stay interested and engaged in being active.

Nix the Temptation to Time It. For several years when I counseled families about incorporating more movement into their day, I'd recommend a specific number of minutes. More often than not, the number made kids and parents feel defeated. While the goal didn't appear overwhelming to me—possibly because I was more open-minded about what constituted beneficial activity—it seemed to lessen their interest in trying to meet it at all. So guess what? I stopped talking about it. Instead of feeling like it doesn't count unless it's a certain number of minutes, focus on how she feels during and after activity and gradually increase the intensity, duration, or skill level of whatever she enjoys week by week. It takes her 30 minutes to walk home from school or to dance through her favorite YouTube video? How about gradually adding time by taking the long way home or adding another song to the playlist? Aim to increase in time (and types of activity) until it's no longer fun or starts interfering with other responsibilities.

INSPIRING MOVEMENT

Some parents tell me their kids just really aren't active. While I tend to believe parents, I also don't recommend they resign themselves to giving up on offering opportunities for movement all together. Some girls might not appear to be athletic, competitive, or fit enough for sports, or graceful or coordinated enough for dance, or curious, energetic, and social enough to be motivated enough to just go outside to run around and play. Yet there's still a good chance that she—like most people—has an innate need to move and a system hardwired to benefit from it emotionally, physically, and, in some situations, socially. She just may need to come to it on her own terms and in her own way.

If you're wondering why I'm so emphatic about the importance of helping your daughter find a way to move that suits her, consider the fact that doing so could help her cope better with just about everything. "During physical activity, muscles secrete hormones into your bloodstream that make your brain more resilient to stress. Scientists call them 'hope molecules,'" explains Stanford research psychologist Kelly

McGonigal, PhD, author of *The Joy of Movement*. Who doesn't want to figure out a way to get your child to secrete more hope molecules?

For girls who are reluctant or less interested in being active, we want to be extra careful to take steps to make sure that our attempts to help our daughter find the kind of movement that feels right for her is always a positive experience. If we don't, we run the risk of spoiling their relationship with physical activity even more. Here are a few pointers to keep the door open for your daughter when it comes to finding the unique type of movement—if any—that she enjoys.

Acknowledge Choice. Weight-inclusive healthcare activist and certified fitness professional Ragen Chastain points out that "a child's relationship with movement will never be a healthy one if it is something they've been forced into. Make sure your daughter understands that she's not obligated to be active and that she has the choice of whether or not to participate at all. This will help her come to the idea of movement completely on her own terms." One way to do this is by giving her access to as many options as possible so she can explore what she likes and doesn't like herself. That doesn't necessarily mean dropping a ton of money on activities, classes, and equipment to just get a taste of it, says Chastain. "So many classes are now available online. If there's something she's interested in, have her try it at home for free on YouTube first, for example."

Allow Quitting. "So many of the adults I work with have had messy breakups with activity and exercise" says Chastain, "and often it started when they were young. Forcing a child to stick out a whole season in a class or on a team that they don't like is no way to develop a lifelong love of movement." Allow your daughter to try something low-risk and make sure she understands that she can quit after five minutes if it doesn't feel right—then emphasize the positive aspects of the situation if she does back out. "There's a joy in quitting. Even if she fails at loving the activity, she's succeeded," says Chastain. "Now she's got more information about herself and knows more about what doesn't feel good and what she doesn't like."

Consider Personality. Just like with food, many of us have certain activity likes and dislikes, temperaments, and personalities. If we can identify them, we can use them to our advantage, particularly if we aren't naturally athletic or interested in movement.

Some of the girls I have worked with swear they hate sports, yet will agree to run around on a soccer field every day after school just because being on the team means extra time with their friends. Some girls brighten up to the idea of walking around the neighborhood or home from school because it gives them some autonomy and independence that they wouldn't otherwise be allowed. Some kids like to move fast, and some prefer to move slowly. Since everyone enjoys movement in their own way, think back to a time when your daughter was moving a lot, say during an impromptu dance session at a birthday party or while at the playground with a few of her friends. Then, see if you can bring those elements forward into something she might like to do regularly, such as signing up for a drumming circle, an obscure type of cultural dance, or having a regular outdoor playdate with a neighborhood friend.

Cut Down on Tech Time. The more minutes spent on screens, the fewer movements we make throughout the day. One lab study even measured a decrease in metabolism when we're in the trancelike state that comes with vegging out in front of a screen.[12] If we put hard limits on phone, tablet, laptop, and television use, there's a good chance our daughters will move more without us even having to mention it. According to another study, when parents cut back on television in particular, their kids were more active, even when they chose other sedentary habits like reading or crafts.[13]

And, yes, I get it! Cutting back on screen time feels tough, especially when there's lots of pushback and the possibility of you having to come up with an alternative source of entertainment. Try using a gradual approach to cutting back, set the same goal for yourself, and be honest and empathetic with your daughter about the fact that this is something you—and many other people—are also struggling with. Focus on the many benefits (i.e. less stress, better sleep, better mood, and better family relationships) to remind you both that it's worth it.

Put Activity on Autopilot. Straight from the science of habit creation, a tactic I recommend parents use and teach their daughters to rely on, too, is to automate daily physical activity or regular movement. For girls who enjoy organized activities such as sports, sign up for a team or class and schedule it on your own calendar just like you would any other priority, which will give you both much less reason to do the daily debate about whether or not you have time or need to do it on any given day, and instead, just get to it. If classes and teams aren't your daughter's thing, get creative about other ways to automate a little movement into her day. For example, forfeiting the bus for biking, scootering, or walking to school.

Encourage Being Outside. If she's not up for a regularly-scheduled activity, simply opening up the door and insisting she spend at least some of her day outside can be enough to make a difference. Girls who spend time outdoors move their bodies significantly *more* than those who tend to spend more free time inside—regardless of what activities they're doing.[14] In other words, your daughter doesn't necessarily need to be signed up for a sport or physical activity to benefit from the fresh air and increased space. Childhood play advocate, researcher, and cognitive development expert Jody DeVos, Ph.D. suggests taking a family stroll after dinner, using stargazing or plant-identifying apps to explore constellations or flora, or simply giving her some chalk so she can draw some art or start a game of hopscotch or foursquare on the driveway or sidewalk.[15]

Create Opportunity without Pressure. To avoid what happened to Mirabel, you can use a division of responsibility approach, similar to what was recommended in Chapter 6 with eating.[16] As parents, we offer daughters regular and consistent opportunities to be physically active in a safe environment. We choose those activities based on whatever resources we have, be it by bringing her to the playground, buying or renting her a bike, inviting her on a walk, signing her up for a sport or class (with her buy-in, of course), or simply making time for her to be outside.

During those activities, we allow her to decide how much or how little she'll move, as well as whether she'll do it at all. We resist the urge to pressure her by having certain expectations for performance or impact on her body or weight, as well as being accepting of her personal level of enjoyment in specific activities (such as soccer, don't ask me how I know). Our disapproval about her performance or level of enthusiasm can discourage her from participating, as well as decrease her belief in her physical ability altogether.

INCREASING COMFORT & SAFETY

Occasionally, I've had clients with larger bodies (or their mothers) tell me that they're not comfortable being active because of their size. If you suspect this is an issue for your daughter, take time to talk to her about it. "If she does want to be active, it's important to drill down on exactly what's getting in her way," says Chastain, who has been a competitive dancer and holds the Guinness World Record for being the heaviest woman to complete a marathon, "that way you can address it." If you have a large chest, it can be physically uncomfortable to run, for example, says Chastain. In these cases, compression clothing can help stop movement and make them more comfortable." If the discomfort is psychological, if they're worried that they're going to be body shamed, for example, "then I think it's important to tell kids openly and honestly that it's not in their heads. Weight stigma is real." To help normalize their own bodies, Chastain recommends sharing examples of folks online who are in larger bodies and doing sports. "The idea that bodies that jiggle during movement may seem wrong to your daughter and make her embarrassed. Showing her other girls and women who jiggle and are doing sports can help her feel more comfortable."

If your daughter complains of discomfort due to limited mobility, you can search online for adaptive or modified movements for plus-size or larger bodies. And regardless of size, if your daughter complains of shortness of breath (due to asthma or another reason) or pain, be sure to have a weight-inclusive medical professional assess the problem. Together you can come up with a safe way to incorporate activity if she gets the all-clear and is interested.

Lastly, reassure your daughter that body size is not an indicator of how strong or capable a person is and physical activity and movement looks and feels different for everyone.

CONNECTING WITH YOUR DAUGHTER THROUGH MOVEMENT

I never understood my mother's obsession with walking, though I was grateful for it. Every early morning around 7:00 a.m., I knew exactly where to find her. Whether it was 90 degrees or two feet of snow, she'd lace up her sneakers, leash up the dog, and head out for a two-mile walk that encompassed our tiny neighborhood. She claimed she was doing it for the series of dogs that were in and out of her house, but even after the last chocolate Labrador went to live with my brother, her daily early morning walks persisted. It's now, in my forties, that I finally understand the importance of simply moving—not fast, not calorie-burning, strengthening, or toning—just putting my body in motion. As her daughter, I had my own reason for considering her habit important—tagging along on those walks was the only place where my mother and I really connected.

In the event that you're feeling distant from your daughter, movement may help bring you back together. When we're physically active with our daughters, we're engaging in something called social motion. If you've ever walked, run, biked, or rowed alongside someone else for some time, you've probably experienced the bonding benefits. You both benefit from the boost in feel-good hormones that come along with any physical activity. In addition, engaging in a physically exerting activity alongside someone else changes brain waves, increasing feelings of cooperation and connection.[17]

As a bonding tip, when you suggest you and your daughter get moving together, be sure to tell her you enjoy her company or simply want to spend time with her, as opposed to focusing on the physical perks of you both being active and, if possible, choose something that will make your bodies move, at least somewhat, in a synchronized manner.

"To connect with our bodies is to learn to trust ourselves, and from that comes power.

—*Mirka Knaster, Discovering the Body's Wisdom*

CENTERING OURSELVES WITH MOVEMENT

I was in 3rd or 4th grade, running laps inside a small Catholic school auditorium when my gym teacher threw me an anchor that I've been latching onto for decades since. As I came around the corner towards the waxy wood stairs of the stage, she jumped in stride alongside me and said, "I really like how you're pacing yourself." *Pacing myself?* All I knew was that I'd given up trying to race the other kids in mindless circles around the perimeter of the small room since I realized there was no telling when this would end. Even still, I was gasping for air.

She continued jogging beside me and I began to wonder if I was in trouble. Then, she went on, "In through your nose, out through your mouth. Control your breath." At some point, I realized she wanted me to do it, was waiting even to hear it. I closed my mouth and took an inhale up through my nostrils. Then I pushed everything out, my lips rounded as if I trying to whistle. It was hard between gasps of breath, and didn't make sense. She told me to slow down my steps a bit as I tried the inhales and exhales again and again. Finally, she left me to get back off at her stop, the stage.

The next time I came around the bend, she was looking right at me. She had long, shiny auburn hair pulled back in a tight ponytail, a stainless-steel whistle hanging from her neck, and a royal-blue track-suit, making her the only person walking our halls without a nun's habit or uniform. As far as I remember, that was the exact way she looked every single day for the six years I went to that school. I puffed up my chest and took a deep inhale like she'd showed me, then exhaled through visibly rounded lips until our eyes broke. Then I heard her yell, "Pace yourself, kids! Watch how Amelia's doing it!" I felt it in my body; I was not the desperate and defeated girl I had been just a few laps ago. She'd given me something to grab onto, to hold. I was no longer self-conscious, but conscious of my embodied self, my breathing, my feet on the floor, my arms moving through the air—not what it *looked like*, simply *how it felt*. And to stay tuned into this magnificent place, I had to tune out everything else.

Nearly forty years later, I still grab hold of that anchor. While I never became a fast or talented runner, I did continue to run. Running saved me from drowning in emotional overwhelm; it forced me to tune everything else out, to pull back into my body, and focus on nothing but the most essential part of being—my breath. When our breath is involved, movement can calm the nervous system, creating a feeling of safety and restoring confidence.[18] If you're anxious, worried, or afraid and hyper-focused on a problem, fast-paced physical activity can ease worries, boost energy, and stop paralyzing rumination.[19] If you're intent on being active to get that kind of emotional relief, you will need to eat.

If you're intent on eating so you can be active, you will start to listen to your body even more closely so you know which foods and how much will work. When I returned to running in my late 20s, those necessary elements of being active were the catalysts that solidified my breakup with dieting for good.

With that experience in mind, I think giving our daughters the opportunities and encouragement they need to discover a type of movement that they can use as an anchor when their worlds become a sea of change or stress is a huge gift, one that will pay back in dividends throughout life. You can use movement as a way to reroute her attention to how her body feels, not how it looks. If you're available to be active alongside her or can talk to her either before or after, you can strengthen this effect even more by encouraging her to cue into her body sensations before, during, and after the activity; for example, by asking her questions about her energy level, muscle tension or tightness, physical pain, emotions, thirst, hunger, and breathing. Then encourage her to care for her body by respecting what it needs. A dry mouth may need water, achy muscles may need a stretch, breathlessness may signal a need to slow down, a racing mind may need you to speed up, and fatigue may be a signal that it's time to rest. Ultimately, she'll be able to employ this habit of honoring the body, not just during movement, but in all times and as second nature.

MOVEMENT FOR GIRLS TO EXPLORE

Certainly, if it gets her body moving and she enjoys it, then it counts as a nourishing form of physical activity! That includes swinging across the monkey bars, dancing to TikTok videos, and cruising to school on her bike. To get the best benefits, aim to keep her engaged in activity regularly and consistently. To help her identify a type of movement she enjoys and can turn to for healing and inner strength now and for years to come, below are some insights on different forms to explore. Remember, it may take some trial and error before she figures out what feels right for her. Being patient and focusing on the positive—she's learning about herself with every try—will up the chances she continues exploring long enough to find something she really enjoys. Activity ideas to try:

Running. While any aerobic (i.e., heart pumping) activity can quell anxiety and protect against depression, running is especially alluring because it can be done almost anywhere, requires little to no equipment, can be done alongside a team or individually, can be incorporated into other activities such as sports, and is easy to continue throughout life. Running can be particularly good for those of us who have a lot of racing thoughts because the repetitive motion of the feet hitting the ground calms the nervous system. Running can be done fast or slow. While running can be intimidating for adults, I've found that girls are much more apt to jump in, especially if it's incorporated into a game or social activity. If you think your daughter would benefit from and need support, look for a local running club. And if running feels too strenuous or overwhelming, start with walking and gradually incorporate short bursts of jogging.

Dance. This type of activity is a bit of a double-edged sword. It's popular among girls who are often eager to participate, classes are easy to find, and it's done to music, which can have its own positive impact on energy, mood, and motivation. Additionally, some forms of dance can be very accepting of bodies that have otherwise been marginalized due to size or shape. However, some forms of dance can be very body-focused and performance is evaluated based on looks and unnatural aesthetics, as opposed to connecting with natural rhythms and movement. Therefore, we need to be careful when selecting the types of dance we give our daughters a chance to explore as well as continue to check in with them when it comes to how the activity is impacting their body esteem.

Similar to gymnastics, or even working out in a gym, wearing tight clothing while executing movement in front of a mirror can contribute to body checking and comparison with peers. If your daughter loves dance, you might consider participating in cultural dance that includes traditional costumes, dances that are performed in a circle with people facing each other, ballroom dance (which is rarely based on physical evaluation and instead on mastering steps), or other forms of dance where there's more clothing such as hip-hop's baggy sweats, tops, and shirts. You can also capitalize on the benefits of music by adding it to other activities such as indoor cycling, running on a treadmill, and walking.

Yoga. Thanks to the fact that it increases body connection and awareness and emphasizes recognizing and respecting one's own feelings and needs, yoga is regarded as a tool in eating disorder recovery. It has been shown as an effective method for improving self-image and alleviating body dissatisfaction, particularly for adolescent and teenage girls.[20]

Martial Arts. Non-competitive forms such as Aikido and Tai Chi have been shown to help kids with emotional regulation and increase self-confidence.

Team Sports. There's something about working together on a team that I think is extra valuable for adolescent and teenage girls. While there was plenty of social drama during those years, I still regularly have dinner with a group of girls that I played soccer with. I'm certain working together on a team is what helped our relationships weather all kinds of storms. Research links team sports with increased protection against depression, less social isolation, increased academic scores, and better moods.[20] Additionally, girls participating in team sports during early adolescence had higher self-esteem three years later. One caveat: sports where she's moving most of the time work best, so inquire about what's going on in practice if it's not already clear. Team sports that involve moderate to vigorous activity that meets daily recommendations (60 minutes) had significantly higher impacts.

Exotic or Recreational Sports. Activities that require seasonal weather, traveling, or significant gear such as climbing, hiking, skiing, surfing, and indoor swimming are also beautiful forms of movement that improve strength, physical skills, and emotional resilience. If you're fortunate enough to be able to offer your daughter an opportunity to participate in them regularly, by all means, encourage it! However, if these activities are done infrequently, I do recommend finding an additional source of movement that can be done routinely and consistently (perhaps training for those activities, if that's a motivator) so that your daughter always has an outlet available.

If I could go back to that moment with Mirabel, I would ask her mother to leave the room to ease the tension and lessen expectation. I would ask her if she liked swimming. I would ask her why. I would ask her to tell me what she feels like when she's in the pool and what she feels like when she gets out of it.

If she answered in all the ways that I think she might, I'd tell her the pool was a special place for her, a space to return to when she felt lost or unsure, a place where she could stand in her own power.

I'd tell her she was lucky to have this space, as not every girl does. I'd tell her to protect this space with all her might, as she could rely on it now and forever. I'd ask her how we could make swimming better for her (on a team or off, in a group or solo, in a pool or a lake).

Then I'd tell her that, in my expert opinion, her body weight did not matter. Regardless of the size and shape or her body, swimming would always be her safe place and her superpower. Then I'd ask her to leave the room so I could once again speak with her mother and father.

With Mirabel's parents I'd share that, yes, they were right; swimming had many health benefits for their daughter—and that we had to avoid making weight control be one of them. I'd recommend preserving the experience as a positive one at all costs, which required them both to stop talking about how good it was for her body shape and, instead, stay silent and do their best to continue to give her an opportunity to do it. Now, whenever "a Mirabel" comes to see me, I am prepared.

REFLECTIONS ON MOVEMENT

- *What is your attitude toward movement? Is it one of play and fun or obligation?*

- *What is your daughter's attitude about movement?*

- *If your daughter avoids movement or does it out of a desire to lose weight, what is one way you can help reframe her attitude towards it?*

- *If your daughter struggles to incorporate movement into her life, what is getting in the way? (For example, self-esteem, fear of being seen, fear of not being good at different activities, lack of space, lack of time?) What is one way you could address this barrier?*

- *If it isn't possible for you and your daughter to be active together at this time, can you be accepting of that? How might that help her?*

CHAPTER TEN
BODY

"Stop trying to fix your body, it was never broken."

—*V, (formerly Eve Ensler)*

A STRUGGLE TO LOVE OUR BODIES IS OFTEN WHAT DRIVES US TO dieting. When we are lucky enough to finally awaken from that misguided endeavor, our ability to cultivate and sustain a deep, generous love for our bodies is the work we are faced with next. Long after we've healed our relationship with food, long after we've changed our approach to feeding our own daughters, long after we've acknowledged that bias against larger bodies is wrong, what often still remains is the impulse to criticize the body we have or lament the body we don't. When we are dedicated to helping our daughters love their own bodies, the persistent grip of our own negative body image can leave us all the more ashamed. The mothers I've worked with have taught me that the lingering struggle for full body love is more normal than not. While getting themselves and their girls on the right track with food is a surprisingly manageable fete, feeling at home in their bodies is something mothers want to keep talking about long after their feeding struggles with their children no longer exist. Whether the hurts are perpetrated by others or self-inflicted, whether they are significant and public or private and seemingly inconsequential, the conversations about struggling to accept the body linger on and on.

It makes sense to me. Despite knowing where I fall in the context of the larger picture of body oppression, despite knowing the risks I might cause my own daughter if I don't "get it together" and start accepting myself as I am, I'd be lying if I said I'm succeeded at putting my own body loathing to rest. Body image can be notoriously difficult to shift. In fact, it's often the last area where women see healing and improvement on the trajectory of eating disorder recovery.

Yet, there may be good news for us as mothers. According to researchers, it is much easier to build positive feelings about our bodies right from the start—rather than bouncing back out of dissatisfaction. And a positive body image is protective against dieting, disordered eating, and eating disorders.[1] Our active awareness of the importance of cultivating a positive body image—not longing for an idolized body size—may make us better able to focus our efforts for our daughters in the right place. Actively working to ensure our girls embrace their physical selves as an incredible part of their being means they'll be much less likely to ever get stuck in that dark space of body discontent nor have to work hard to fight their way out of it.

With this in mind, instead of feeling like a fraud for preaching body acceptance to our daughters while inwardly cringing at the size of our thighs, we can remind ourselves that we're not alone in our struggle, nor is there anything uniquely imperfect about our body in particular. With some insight, patience, and understanding, our body appreciation can and will blossom and grow. And doing so won't just be the last leg of our own journey in coming to a happy, healthy place with food and body. If we are wrestling with our reflection in the mirror ourselves, it can serve as a powerful and necessary reminder of all those dark feelings and dieting trauma we're fighting to protect our daughters from.

THE BODY PROBLEM

Certainly, there are multiple reasons that body dissatisfaction is so persistent and resistant to change, and often the last thing we recover in our battle to put our weight and eating issues to rest. Girls as young as three have reported being concerned about the way their body looks, perhaps because we internalize the thin ideal at such an early age. Even when we've mended our own wounds from diet culture, the constant agitation of the media's messages prevents us from ever fully healing. As women, we've been trained to *see* our bodies instead of experience them, constantly considering how we look instead of how we feel. Even the term *body image* is what Elizabeth Scott LCSW, CEDS-S, co-founder of The Body Positive calls "fundamentally dissociative" since it triggers us to focus "on how we are seen from outside of ourselves," which is most often "through the eyes of a critical, judging authority."

MAKING BODY LOVE THE NORM

Not liking our bodies is the default reaction for the majority of us. It was such an obvious phenomenon, in fact, that in the 1980s researchers began referring to it as "normative discontent." And many of us have grown up in a culture that just expects us to be unhappy with our bodies and, in the case of marketers, they prey on it.

However, more recently, eating disorder researchers have explained that actively rejecting the notion that body hate is normal is an important way to help reverse the trend, especially for those most at risk for developing issues such as girls.[2] In other words, making sure our daughters don't assume that being unhappy with their body or their weight is just part of being a girl, a rite of passage, or even an issue to bond over (as in in the tendency for an "I feel fat" comment to universally get a "me, too!" response), can make them more resilient against ever developing body dissatisfaction in the first place. And that's important because once it sets in, this particular kind of discontent can be tough to recover from. In other words, calling out body self-loathing as wrong, unproductive, and unhealthy from the beginning is a more effective approach than waiting until we pick up on their own body unhappiness and then trying to correct it. When I hear others putting their bodies down or dissecting perceived flaws in shape or size with my daughters as witnesses, I regard it as nothing short of absurd—and I make no bones about saying so. *Bodies are amazing. Your body did nine million different things right, just to get you here today, including pumping blood to a bazillion microscopic cells, firing off neurons and contracting muscles, helping you walk, talk, smile, and even understand what I'm saying to you right now. How could you ever regard it as anything less than incredible?* (More on body appreciation, my favorite method to increasing body love, later in this chapter.)

First and foremost, above overcorrecting other people's negative body talk, I suggest never letting a putdown your daughter expresses about her own body go unaddressed. Even if it sounds familiar, normal, or innocent, taking a moment to question or challenge a comment from your daughter can go a long way in subverting the feeling that we're obliged to hate our body, looks, shape, or weight.

A few suggestions for making the conversation positive and productive that I recommend to my clients may help. First, always *lead with gratitude*. Being thankful when she shares feelings with you, even if they are tough to hear, can make sure that the door between the two of you stays open. Second, *be curious*: our daughters' experiences are their own, so it's best to avoid assumptions which can lead to misunderstandings. Instead, ask, "What makes you say that?" or "What makes you feel that way?" and let her fill you in on the details as she sees them. Be honest and factual, as opposed to giving your opinion when responding to her concerns. You might note, for example, that you can't *feel* fatness. Fat is a physical thing not an emotional state of being, such as feeling happy, sad, or surprised. (What she is feeling is probably more like self-judgment, dislike, or a feeling of failure for not living up to what society considers a social norm or the thin ideal.) However, you do have fat on your body—everyone does. And, yes, your body is different from hers and others—no two bodies are the same. Be *empathetic* by recognizing that not meeting ideals can feel hard, yet that doesn't mean her body is wrong, unhealthy, or incorrect. And the self-judgment is neither necessary nor warranted.

Finally, avoid telling her that the way she feels about her body is unnecessary or untrue. Don't deny her experience. For example, when my daughter told me she "felt fat" while getting ready for dance class, my instinct was to respond, "No, you're not!" I stop myself from saying this as often as I can—not only to my daughter but to my clients, friends, and anyone else who insists such a thing in front of me. The reason? Acknowledging anti-fat bias and pointing it out as harmful or wrong gives her a better shot at dealing with it in a positive, productive way. Second, responding by focusing your attention on her body size and shape and what *you* think about it can reinforce the idea that you think these things are important as well as minimize her feelings. Lastly, insisting that she isn't fat implies that being fat is a terrible, no good, very bad thing, which it isn't. Being in a larger body or having fat on your body is not the scary, horrible thing that we're being conditioned to think it is—and it certainly isn't as bad as harm dieting may do to her.

In addition, there's a very good chance that her body may one day be fatter than it is now, and we want her to be indifferent to those changes rather than wage war against them. Neutralizing the fear of fat will lessen the pressure to conform to unrealistic standards. And further, remember that her complaints are not actually about how much fat she does or doesn't have on her body, so there's no use in arguing that. It's about how she *feels* about her body, and we need her to be able to process negative feelings towards her body shape in a positive way, instead of telling her she shouldn't have them.

EMBRACING EMBODIMENT

One blistering cold Sunday morning, I was running a recreational race in Central Park when I realized that the icy cold sting on my skin of my right hip was happening for a good reason. Thanks to a super-fast exit from a porta-potty, pre-race, the waistband of my leggings was twisted and scrunched down, revealing a chubby flank of skin exposed to the wind. Mortified, I unraveled it, stretched it up as high as it could go, pulled my many layers of shirts down on top, and smoothed the whole situation with the palm of my hand. I'd slowed my pace and weaved in and out of other runners to become anonymous in the crowd once again.

What could the people behind me have been thinking about my muffin-top? And can they see the bumpy cellulite on the back of my legs? At that moment, the word *self-objectification* came hurling through the air, smacking me right in the face. "Self-objectification is the invisible prison of picturing yourself being looked at instead of just fully living," explains Lindsay and Lexie Kite, PhDs in *More Than a Body: Your Body is an Instrument, Not an Ornament.* Once I started worrying about how I looked from behind, I was no longer a runner. I was an object to be seen.

Recognizing and rejecting the objectification of women is important work, yes! Seeing how women are depicted as objects to be looked at, as opposed to persons who are just *being*; and understanding that it is wrong is so helpful for our daughters. More importantly, we need to also understand how we objectify ourselves, seeing our bodies as opposed to being in them. This is an area where we have control. When I see my reflection in a storefront mirror and wince at how round I am, I'm self-objectifying. When I skip out on jumping in the town pool with my girls because I'm worried about what my neighbors might think about my weight, I'm limiting my life by thinking about how I look to others instead of living. I can actively catch myself and step out of that self-inflicted prison by rejecting the impulse to see myself as an image being viewed by an outside authority. If we notice our daughters building a prison around themselves, bar by bar, self-image by self-image, we can reject it as par for the course and suggest she stop inflicting that same critique—good or bad, positive or negative—about how she looks instead of how she feels.

Alternatively, focusing on how you feel in your body, or embodiment, can counter self-objectification and be empowering. "Embodiment guides us to the subjective experience of how it feels to live inside our bodies and to identify with our own unique experience," explains Scott. If it is possible for your daughter to do it, physical activities that are fast-paced or require coordination or concentration are particularly effective as ways to recenter ourselves in our body and enjoy that sweet freedom of just being, as opposed to being seen. It's not an ironic coincidence that my own personal epiphany on this particular matter occurred while running: I think it was the fact that I was so very much in my body that when I was taken out of it, the jarring contrast in my mood and mindset was so stark that I couldn't help but wake up to the difference between the freedom of moving, breathing, and being in my body compared to the paralytic experience of envisioning myself being seen.

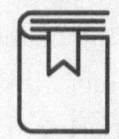

Bookmark If you want to do a deep dive into the topic as well as get more tips on recognizing and overcoming it in your own life, head straight to *Chapter 3. From Self-Objectification to Self-Actualization* in *More Than a Body* by Lindsay Kite. PhD, and Lexie Kite, PhD.

NORMALIZING FAT & PUBERTY

As women, our body changes throughout life again and again and again. Hormonal changes—such as puberty, pregnancy, menopause, aging, and changes during times of stress—cause shifts in our appetite, energy use, and fat storage. A changing body is normal and healthy. The sooner we help our daughters to understand and accept a changing body as a fact of being human—instead of bracing themselves against it—the better.

Puberty is one of the first times our girls will encounter dramatic and visual body changes. When our girls (and the adults around them) are unprepared for those changes, a rounding tummy is much more likely to cause alarm. In fact, if we ourselves have latent fears about fatness or a past history of trauma with food or dieting, then our girls' changing bodies might trigger our own issues. We, too, need to reassure ourselves that all is well and normal, otherwise we might search for ways to pump the brakes on her increased eating, appetite, or weight. Of course, as we've learned in earlier chapters, restriction is the enemy, as it leads to a multitude of other negative impacts on lifelong eating and body image. Instead, reminding ourselves and our daughters that increases in body fat and a changing shape just prior to and during puberty are normal and necessary can help quell fears and preserve a happy, healthy relationship with food.

Right up there with talking to her about her impending period, bringing up the fact that a female body tends to put on some extra fat during preadolescent, adolescent, tween, and teen years can go a long way in helping her feel at ease about it. Boys' bodies, for example, get leaner during puberty, with overall fat mass decreasing, while girls' overall fat mass does just the opposite, gradually increasing from puberty to early adulthood. Aim for matter-of-factness about the changes themselves—and there's no need to get into the numbers—as well as the reasons for the changes. You can also emphasize how incredible the body is for knowing exactly what to do, which can go a long way when it comes to curing the impulse to rage against changes by dieting.

I also recommend opening the door and inviting her to talk about how these changes might make her feel. While we don't want to normalize body loathing, we can normalize feeling weird or uncomfortable about the transformation. This understanding can go a long way in helping her be more self-compassionate if she's struggling, as well as more accepting of the body she's growing into. This conversation can also be an opportunity to reframe the changes as a sign that her body is healthy and doing exactly what it is meant to do, not something that we need to fight against.

Another reason that your adolescent daughter might be very vulnerable to body image disturbances is that often she is dealing with body changes right around the time she's moving from elementary to middle school, which can mean a change in environment, routine, and even peer group. Plus, your daughter's increase in body fat will be a stark contrast to what the males she knows are going through, since their overall fat mass is simultaneously decreasing (and more in line with cultural ideals of thinness), which could make her own changes feel all the more conflicting.

Further, a body that's becoming more woman than girl may cause girls to feel like they're being viewed differently by family or those whom they've known for a long time. Puberty was traumatic for me—and I'm going to go out on a limb and assume that it was for you, too. Everyone around me seemed uncomfortable that I was no longer the cute little girl of the family and was instead, a full-chested woman (or looked like one, at least), and I felt blame. Never underestimate how difficult this time in your daughter's life may be, nor how tempting dieting to fend off body changes might seem as a way to stabilize the unwanted turbulence.

FINDING COMFORT IN CLOTHING

After I earned my graduate degree, I had an opportunity to join a friend in working with a multi-level marketing (MLM) company for women's athleisurewear. Of course, it was an overall disaster with the exception of one bright shining light which came in the form of an annual company-wide conference. I flew with a friend to Kentucky to attend, and while there, I listened to an incredible speaker who, in an effort to get us excited about getting other women excited about buying clothing, got me thinking a whole lot about how looking in my closet made me feel. I kid you not; I flew home intrigued with a new awareness of all the emotion that was happening every time I contemplated my collection of clothing.

As it turns out, those three pairs of jeans that hadn't fit since the year before my daughter was born, those expensive wool pants I still couldn't button, and the stretchy tanks that kept doing that uncomfortable roll up thing seemed to fill me with sadness, fear, hostility, frustration, and hopelessness. Heavy, right? On the other hand, the stretchy jeans and soft, oversized sweater, well they made me feel happy, safe, and accepted. So what did I do to ratchet up good vibes? I got rid of every single thing that did not fit and with that also erased about several thousand unnecessary moments of self-inflicted body shame. Do I have a lot less clothing? Yes, and those losses have been so worth it. I invite you to liberate yourself from the same closet shame and extend that gift to your daughter, too.

Of course, it can be challenging to keep up with her changing size without interfering in what she does and does not want to wear. Yet when it comes to checking in on how things fit, I wouldn't underestimate its importance. With her help, identify things that no longer fit and get rid of them sooner rather than later, which can lessen the odds she'll be making deals with herself about how to get back into them. You can also remove size tags, as well as have a conversation about how inaccurate and inconsistent those numbers can be if she's focusing on them. I suggest emphasizing the importance of the functionality of clothing and how things feel rather than how they look when choosing clothing.

BEING MINDFUL ABOUT BODY TALK

Speaking of clothing, I was never more aware of how harshly I could nitpick my own appearance than when I entered a Lord & Taylor fitting room with my six-year-old to find a dress for a cousin's wedding. Knowing full well she was raptly watching and listening, I had to bite my tongue on every body-centered criticism that crossed my mind. It was a fairly silent 20 minutes. And even while I remained mum, the looks on my face threatened to betray me. For a person who was ready to pounce when others put their bodies down, my own inner critic was being fiercely disobedient. Color, creativity of the designer (I was grasping for straws), and whether or not I'd be cold were the only comments, considerations, and laments that I let my daughter hear from me.

If you're reading this book, you already know your daughter isn't only listening to friends and media; she's listening to you, too. What you might not know is that, as mothers, our reflexive disapprovals (spoken or unspoken) about our own body are especially contagious. Girls who sense their mother is dissatisfied with her body are more likely to be dissatisfied with their own body, regardless of its shape and size.[3] If you're like me, setting the intention to avoid talking about your own body might serve as a wakeup call to just how often, unkind, and mindlessly you might be doing it.

In addition, I've found it helpful to make it clear to my daughter that we don't talk about the way other people's bodies look, either. (Compliments about function and skill—like a runner with strong legs or a dancer who moves with grace, are welcome, especially if the person has worked hard to earn it. Making judgements about the way someone's body looks? Not okay. As they get older, girls will better understand the nuances.) In addition, I make my girls and all my clients very clear on the fact that a person isn't fat; they "have fat" on their body, and we cannot tell how healthy or unhealthy a person is by the way their body looks. Both ideas can reinforce the positive regard for their own physique.

Furthermore, weight-based teasing, in particular, whether it's done at school or at home, is especially harmful to body image, and increases the risk for depression and eating disorders, making it an urgent place to step in. Some research shows that adolescents experiencing this problem really want their parents' support. And of course, helping her lose weight—even if that's the kind of support she's asking for—isn't an effective way to do it. Instead, help her build self-acceptance with the tips shared in Chapter 7.

• •

ENCOURAGING BODY APPRECIATION

When it comes to talking to your daughter, you can start by redirecting her attention to the things her body does for her—its function—whenever she makes a comment about how she looks. If you already practice gratitude with your daughter, you can slip feeling thankful about your body into that as well. For younger girls, you might try saying, "I'm so lucky," as opposed to "I'm grateful for" or "I really appreciate." And you can throw out those comments whenever you see fit. If you're feeling stumped, here are a few examples to get started:

- We're so lucky we have strong legs that we can use to peddle these bikes, walk us to school, run across that whole field, ski a mountain, or climb a hill.

- I'm really grateful for my eyes—they're working every day to help me read, watch this movie, see the sunset, and let me know if it's safe to cross the street.

- Isn't our heart amazing? It's pumping blood through our whole body all day and night without us even thinking about it.

- Your fingers are awesome! They helped you weave this basket, write this story, and figure out which avocado was ripe enough to eat.

- Your arms are so strong! I can't believe you carried all those things at once, swung that bat so hard, pulled yourself up on those bars, and played the piano for ten minutes straight.

- Your body is amazing! It's growing exactly the way it is supposed to.

- Your tummy is brilliant! It knows out to break up all the foods we eat and turn them into fuel so our body can have energy, grow, build bones, build muscles, learn, and think.

- Body appreciation is one of a growing number of concepts, practices, and social movements dedicated to helping people (women, primarily) improve how they relate to their own bodies. To learn more about the difference between body resilience, body appreciation, body positivity, weight inclusivity, weight neutrality, fat acceptance, fat activism, and more, as well as how to connect with these movements and how they might each help your daughter improve her relationship with her body, visit NourishHer.com/body-movements.

• •

PRACTICING SOCIAL MEDIA SELF-CARE

Several months before writing this chapter, a terrifying moment during a workshop hosted by a well-known eating disorder center took my breath away. It was right after the presenter reviewed research on the impacts of social media use, including increases in body dissatisfaction, drive for thinness, disordered eating, eating concerns, anxiety, and depression. She went on to explain the responsive and ever-evolving technology, called collaborative or social filtering, that made apps such as TikTok and Instagram particularly harmful and addictive, and it hit me—*What if the women's magazines I was so infatuated with as a tween and teen could have been adaptive and responsive to my 15-year-old self?*

I imagined, for a moment, opening one of my favorite magazines to an advertisement featuring Kate Moss, a bony, hipless, waifish model well-known for posing half naked in men's underwear. What if the magazine sensed me lingering on that image, then changed all the pages that followed to feature more and more girls who looked the same? What if it responded to me reading workouts about getting thinner thighs or erasing cellulite by filling every one of the following pages with more diet tips, tricks, and cheats to keep me focused on more of the same?

My obsessions would've been reinforced, insecurities heightened, and worse, I'd miss out on being exposed to alternative images, topics, or points of view. I wouldn't have turned to an essay by a young woman who'd overcome an eating disorder and become skeptical of the safety of my dieting, nor that life-changing article on dysthymia that finally helped me recognize and get help for my depression. If I had had responsive media in my back pocket and on-demand as a teenager, the consequences on my body image (and more!) would've been devastating. It's no wonder that social media use is associated with heightened body dissatisfaction for girls, as well as increased depression and anxiety, and a lower overall quality of life.[4]

Despite the knowledge that social media use among children can be harmful, I do accept that it is part of many girls' social reality and believe it's our responsibility as parents to give them the tools to use it responsibly. Girls between ages 11 and 13 are particularly vulnerable to the impacts of social media, thanks, in part, to their developmental stage and hormonal changes, With this vulnerability in mind, it's integral to put measures for self-care protection in place during or before that time. In my opinion, if your daughter is old enough to have access to social media—even on someone else's device and without her own account, then she's old enough to learn how to enjoy these apps while also protecting herself from possible harm. And there are positives such as free education, exposure to body diversity, anti-diet information (you may not know about this book if it weren't for social media, for example), encouraging self-care, and decreasing stigmatization or loneliness with access to new communities. For those who do use social media, be mindful about use and avoid mindlessly scrolling. Here are more tips that can help you and your daughter use social media positively:

SOCIAL MEDIA SELF-CARE PLAN OF ACTION

First, start by having a conversation—the start of many ongoing conversations—about the purpose of her device. Explain that while it can help entertain, inspire, connect, and educate, it can also be a source of negativity. It can be a distraction, an annoyance, a time-waster, a source of irritation, and can cause self-criticism. Explain that it's important to make sure her device is helping and making her life better—not worse.

Second, ask her about the purpose of the device in her own life. Why did she get it and why does she need it? Was it meant to entertain her, to inspire, to connect with her friends, to educate? Write her reasons down in a place you can both see. Once you are solid on the purposes, go through each app on the device and delete those that don't meet one or more of those reasons. You might even go as far as creating a contract outlining your agreed-upon expectations for how your daughter will use a device. Teens and media expert Ana Homayoun calls this an *Acceptable Use Media Agreement*. She recommends parents collaborate with their children to decide what goes in the contract and touch on three key areas, including how they will self-regulate use (aka limit time spent), handle social issues, and be safe.

Next, together you can open up each of the social media apps she uses, such as Instagram, Facebook, and TikTok. For each app, look at the individual accounts she follows, asking *What do you like about this account? How does looking at this person's posts make you feel?* Take time to sit with her and really listen as she talks about her feelings. She may be ambivalent at first, and it could take time for her to get insight into exactly how she's feeling. It may be difficult for her to be critical of other accounts, especially if they are peer accounts. Suggest she delete any accounts that aren't serving one of her original purposes or that make her feel down or sad. If she's reluctant, ask her to talk about the benefits of keeping them—as well as the benefits of deleting them. If accounts are about fitness, health, or eating, encourage her to go deeper about what she views as "healthy" and avoid letting that be a blanket reason for focusing on these topics in particular. Use information you learned earlier in this book to help her be more discerning about whether accounts are really keeping her well emotionally, socially, and physically.

Finally, an important skill to give your daughter is the ability to distinguish what is real and what isn't. This kind of discernment is found in women who are less burdened by emotional stress from social media. For example, in further sessions with Mirabel she kept lamenting that her "tummy wasn't flat enough." As we talked more about why that mattered to her, she shared photos of classmates who'd been posting pics of their stomach on Instagram, each thinner than the next. Amongst other things, I pointed out how contorted their poses were, and how unrealistic such an impossibly thin abdomen would be in real life, and asked her what she thought one might have to do to develop a tummy that flat. After she described the grueling, time-consuming, joyless routine and limited diet one would need to adhere to in order to achieve that, she also acknowledged that having such a look wasn't worth the price one needed to pay.

 **Bookmark:** For more actionable steps on managing social media, see Chapter 4: "Conversations: How to Talk to Your Kids About Social Media" in *Social Media Wellness: Helping Tweens and Teens Thrive in an Unbalanced Digital World* by Ana Homayoun. This book contains strategies, real life stories, and tactical tips to help you help your child manage the interaction between their real and virtual lives, including templates of agreements you can make with your daughter about social media use, specific apps for parental control of devices, ideas for lessening social media distractions throughout the day, which, frankly, even most of us adults will find useful!

BODY IMAGE RESILIENCE

As you come up against objectification and reminders of just how rampant body image struggles remain, you can remind yourself that you've already equipped your daughter with a certain body image resiliency. Body image resilience, a term I first learned about from the Kite sisters' book, is our ability to avoid body dissatisfaction regardless of our experience with it. In other words, while we might not be able to wipe the world clean of the tendency to objectify ourselves nor make our girls blind to ever-present images of the thin ideal, we can take steps to lessen the negative impact of those factors on our daughters. Boosting our daughters' body image resilience lowers their risk of body dissatisfaction.[5] You've done this just by reading this book, educating yourself about alternative ways to think about food, eating, and weight, and taking steps to develop your own IFM. In fact, body image resilience is built through having supportive families (that's you, momma!), lessening sociocultural pressures and rejecting the thin ideal, improving our relationship with our physical self, increasing coping skills, and prioritizing wellness.

Simply put, by reading this book you will likely increase your daughter's body image resilience by subtly helping her learn to better care for, trust, and respect her body regardless of what size it is, how it might change, or the circumstances she might face.

REFLECTIONS ON BODY

- *What is one thing you can do to help your daughter be more "in" her body (as opposed to worrying about what it looks like)?*

- *What influences may be harming your daughter's feelings about her body?*

- *What can you do to help minimize these influences?*

- *What influences might improve her feelings about her body?*

- *If you could tell your daughter one thing about your own relationship with your body when you were her again until now, what would it be?*

CHAPTER ELEVEN
BEING KNOWN

"Understand this if you understand nothing:
it is a powerful thing to be seen."

—*Akwaeke Emezi, Freshwater*

MANY NIGHTS AT ABOUT 7:31P.M., WHICH IS ONE MINUTE after Alexa has announced in her semi-robotic voice, "It's-time-to-get-ready-for-bed," one of my daughters will ask my husband or me to put on a song.

My girls love putting on shows, which double as a perfect stall tactic before the mutually dreaded bedtime routine. For the show, they each take turns choosing a song from the latest Disney movie or Taylor Swift album.

I usually stand by the side of the couch to watch and alternate between smiling at them in approval and shouting over the music for them to stop jumping off the furniture. Mostly, I'm hoping it'll end and counting the minutes until I can get them into bed.

A few months ago, I was too lazy to find my phone to get dance time started, so I asked Alexa for 'dance songs.' At some point, "Borderline" by Madonna came on. I must have had a cocktail or glass of wine with dinner, because I immediately got up from the couch, closed my eyes, and started dancing. I was mouthing the words and spinning. It was awesome and energizing and fun, just like it always was. At some point, I opened my eyes and noticed everyone else had stopped. My oldest girl stood, mouth gaping as she stared at me. My husband held his phone in his outstretched arm and appeared to be videotaping me. My littlest dove towards me to bury her face in my leg. That's when I realized that muffled yet familiar voice that had been drowned out in the background was her screaming, "Mommy! Stop! Stop!"

I stopped moving to catch my breath. Aside from my husband, who was perfectly and completely tickled, the room was filled with a sort of unfamiliar gravity. I took a deep breath, rolled my eyes and mouthed to my husband, "What's wrong with them?" I was irritated. I was self-conscious. I was a bit ashamed, and a lot confused.

I ended my discomfort by calling it. "Okay, time for bed!" I signaled in my stern it's-time-to-get-stuff-done voice. Surprisingly, both of the girls quietly acquiesced and made their way up the stairs without protest. They were ready to leave this moment behind them. As I, too, climbed the stairs through strange quiet, it hit me. My joy had really scared them! My daughters were totally and completely rattled by the sight of me having so much fun. They could not comprehend this totally foreign version of their mother. The version of me that was dancing, singing, laughing, and being in the moment—the me that was moving my body in energetic, silly, and unexpected ways. Yet they needed to recognize these other parts of me. For their own well-being *and* mine.

There are so many examples of my real self being hidden from my daughters that I can share, like the time my five-year-old told me, "Just wait here," as she and her father swam towards the part of a lake where you could no longer stand, "since you don't know how to swim." Or the time my eight-year-old coasted alongside me on her bike, smiling from ear to ear, saying she didn't know that I knew how to ride. Had they never seen me put my head under the water or take a few laps just for fun? Had they no idea that I'd once swam a mile in the Hudson, or ridden my bike fifty miles as part of a triathlon? No. No. And nope. Just what was going on? Was their ability to see me very limited? Or was I hiding? Or in becoming their mother, had I in some way erased everything I ever was, could be, or become?

In sharing the idea that my daughters don't recognize me when I'm being myself and having fun, I'm reminded of how badly I'd wanted to know my own mother. I remember how intrigued I was when I found a charm bracelet in her jewelry box. Holding each miniature pewter trinket in my hand, they described a woman who I wanted desperately to meet, a woman who took cruises with girlfriends to the Virgin Islands, dreamed of being an interior designer, won an achievement award from The County Trust, and loved the sound of conga drums. How foreign that young woman was, and how I longed to meet her. Maybe I was more similar to my mother than she'd let me think. Maybe I would have had more to admire her for, to respect her for, than the fact that she'd put her entire life on hold to raise me and my brother—more to emulate in my own life.

This is the reason I invite you to *be known* to your daughter. Maybe you don't necessarily want them to see you a little bit tipsy dancing to a decades-old pop song. Or maybe you do? Maybe she needs to see more than just the *mother* you, but more of the *real* you—your joys and sorrows, dreams and ambitions, successes, mistakes, missteps, and all.

> "Mothers have martyred themselves in their children's names since the beginning of time. We have lived as if she who disappears the most, loves the most. We have been conditioned to prove our love by slowly ceasing to exist. What a terrible burden for children to bear—to know that they are the reason their mother stopped living. What a terrible burden for our daughters to bear—to know that if they choose to become mothers, this will be their fate, too. Because if we show them that being a martyr is the highest form of love, that is what they will become. They will feel obligated to love as well as their mothers loved, after all. They will believe they have permission to live only as fully as their mothers allowed themselves to live."
>
> —*Glennon Doyle, Untamed*

Before we were mothers, we weren't. We just were. Daughters, yes. In some ways, that is hard enough. But mothers, no; not yet. We were so many things that as mothers we are not. So I ask you, *where do all those little pieces of us go? And why do we feel the need to disappear at all?* If you can't listen to me, listen to Glennon. Your daughter needs you to remain being *you*. And if you can't possibly imagine doing it for yourself, then do it for her. In doing so, you give her permission to be herself, too.

At the time that I'm preparing to publish this book, my oldest daughter is on the brink of turning 11. While she has never been interested in me as a nutritionist, her intrigue about me as a writer is palpable. She knows I'm working on a project that's important to me and, once it's out in the world, she'll have to go no further than the title to get an introduction to the problem at hand. She'll be disappointed for sure; she's a die-hard Harry Potter fan and this work has nothing in common with fantasy or fiction. Still, putting this book out into the world means that it'll be necessary to repeat an awkward, uncomfortable talk we've had before. I will remind her what dieting is and why people do it. I will have to remind her of the unjust fact that many people judge others by the size and shape of their body. Since there's nothing worse than opening (and reopening) an innocent, sensitive child's eyes to a cruel reality of the world, I suspect my face will turn red, my ears will get hot, and I will be breathless for a moment. What I will need to tell her for the first time is my own part in the matter. That while I now know dieting is wrong there was a time that I did it myself.

I know there is power in sharing my experience. I know that being honest about my own mistakes, maligned views, and missteps will give her an opportunity to see a larger perspective, permission to feel confused and uncomfortable as well as have the courage and knowledge that despite the pressures she may face, she has the innate ability to rise above them.

More practically speaking, I will avoid sharing the specifics of my eating and not eating behaviors, my ways of purging or starving or otherwise abusing my body. I will avoid sharing numbers of pounds lost and gained and numbers weighed then or now. Those specifics are all as damaging as they are inconsequential. In age-appropriate ways, I will share only the most important parts of my dieting story, which is that I made a grave mistake by thinking I could fix my discomfort in the world by becoming thinner or smaller, by starving or shrinking.

My hope is to embolden both of my girls to reject the notion should they ever feel pressured to diet themselves smaller. I'll do this by teaching them how their own body works, to respect and admire its brilliance in function. I'll encourage them to be accepting of its dysfunction too. I'll teach them what I learned the hard way, the lessons I wish my mother had taught me and her mother had taught her, which are how to listen very carefully to the many languages their body speaks to them. And, equally, how to tune out the voices of those who tell them that their body is wrong.

DEFINING WHAT IT MEANS TO BE SEEN FOR YOURSELF

When this book was just a wee little thing, a glint of light that caught my eye, a tiny little infant that I was nursing and molding and considering, I threw a possible outline onto the shared online board of my writing group. When I jotted the title for this chapter, it was more of a whimsy or a dream than a proven concept or set of skills that I've mastered and feel qualified to preach about. Like many things in my life, it was a wish with no real tangible plan. Yet, I had the nerve to write it into the outline of the book anyway. I'm sure I thought that I could figure it out later, that it'd get cut, or that it'd never come to pass.

Just like so many things I have the courage to throw out into the world when I'm not quite paying attention, something unexpected got tossed back. Almost every mother in the group commented on the title of this chapter with encouraging and expectant comments. "I'm so excited for this one!" one wrote. "Oh my, I need this!" shared another. I was so curious about what they were expecting, what they needed, and of course, what I had intended to address when I came up with the idea.

Two years later, I am confronted with this title again. While I'd love to explain a concept, provide a list of proven benefits, then share a set of instructions for doing it or tell you what works for me, here's the truth: I really don't know how to be known to my daughters. I just don't. I don't even know where to look for that kind of information. The only thing I know is that it's vitally important—and, for some of us, equally difficult—to do it.

Being truly known to your daughter is not selfish or self-validating. When you let your daughter see you as you truly are—your dreams, desires, and ambitions, as well as your fears, insecurities, imperfections, idiosyncrasies, mistakes, and missteps—you also show her that you accept all those parts of yourself. You show her that you are a work in progress. And when she sees you actively standing in that acceptance and eternal quest to evolve, I believe you give your daughter permission to do the same.

Also, I ask not what are the parts you *want* her to see, but also the parts that *need* to be seen? So that one day, if she finds herself mothering someone else, she will know she, too, can remain whole, to simultaneously hold tight to her desires, her dreams, her mistakes, her triumphs, and ambitions without feeling guilty or ashamed or untrue to herself.

Just asking these questions yourself may help you unfurl yourself from the traps of motherhood in a cathartic, meaningful way. You don't need to have an explicit discussion with your daughter about them. You can do this in a private, safe way, such as by sitting quietly with the questions in your mind and stopping when it's uncomfortable. Or writing the answers in a journal or typing them into a document. The key is giving yourself a moment to think about these things, enough to shine light on the you that needs to be known to your daughter and hers, and so on. For your daughter's sake, I hope those sides of you come out when you are ready.

REFLECTIONS ON BEING KNOWN
TO YOUR DAUGHTER

- *What did you wish you knew about your own mother? Who was she before she had you? What were her dreams, interests, values, and passions? Do you know? If you don't, would you like to?*

- *What do you think your mother "gave up" to be a mother?*

- *What is an activity, interest, or passion that you no longer do now that you're a mother?*

- *Would you be interested in starting it again? If so, what would be the benefit to you? What might be the benefit to your daughter?*

CHAPTER TWELVE
RADIATING CHANGE

"Ours is not the task of fixing the entire world all at once, but of stretching out to mend the part of the world that is within our reach…"

—*Clarissa Pinkola Estés, Letter to a Young Activist During Troubled Times: Do Not Lose Heart, We Were Made for These Times*

THE DIFFERENCE BETWEEN BEING A HEALTHY EATER AND A dieter *en route* to a disordered, stressed, and unwell relationship with food is no longer a great chasm but a fine line that is growing ever so faint. Many of us, having crossed that chasm ourselves, know the dangers of going there and want nothing more than to protect our daughters from doing the same.

As mothers and feeders, we have to decide if we are willing to let that line blur further by pushing a thinner-is-better, "healthy" eating agenda—or if we're going to embrace an IFM and darken that line in the sand between extreme and restrictive eating and eating well once again. If we are determined enough, if we are courageous enough, then we can share our own histories with food, our own experiences with limiting and obsessing and starving, not to deepen that line so much as to crack the surface and kick that great divide wide open again. In doing so, we can protect our daughters from losing a part of their life, a part of their deeper self, to the pain and shame of dieting. By embracing an IFM, we offer our daughters a route to reconnect with their appetite, body, and food in positive, nourishing ways. We create an opportunity to see our relationship with them and their relationship with themselves thrive.

With this book in hand, you can now return to the touchstones when challenges come up. When books and blogs and apps promise to help you and your daughter "be a healthy eater," you can discern whether or not their influence is going to help or harm her relationships with body, food, and weight. When your sister-in-law gets wide-eyed when she spots the Cheez-its in your cupboard and tries to help by saying, "Processed foods aren't healthy," you can decide if you think she's right or if agreeing with her and restricting them might destroy your daughter's eating well-being. When your daughter gains some weight and you're worried about how your own mother, the pediatrician, or even your daughter herself might react, you can reassure yourself with knowledge that engaging in a battle with body weight itself is misguided and harmful. When you're wondering whether you should intervene when your daughter reaches for a third scoop of ice cream or whether what feels like a half-bottle of ketchup she's just squeezed onto her plate is good for her, you can lean into trust. You can trust that she is going to be okay. Trust that making mistakes with eating is how we grow. Trust that controlling her decisions about how much she eats or how much she enjoys a food isn't going to serve her well later on.

We also learned the value of our own acceptance when it comes to eating, food, and body, as well as how to communicate with our language and tone. Self-compassion and self-acceptance are gifts we cultivate for our daughters, both of which can improve their self-esteem and overall well-being much more effectively than shame or disapproval. With a new, more simplistic understanding of nutrition, we've come to appreciate just what good eaters our daughters can be (or already are). Our more relaxed approach helps increase their ability to enjoy new foods over time as well as to be more well-nourished. With a new take on physical activity and exercise, we can see movement not as a calorie-burning body sculptor but an intrinsic avenue for developing a positive connection to the body. When we're able to embrace movement as a cathartic path to wholeness, we can increase our daughter's ability to feel good about her physical body irrespective of how it measures up to cultural (and ever-changing) norms.

By going deeper into our own body image issues and our tendency towards objectification, we open up new pathways for understanding when it comes to supporting our daughter's own capacity for embodiment over improving her body image. And by recognizing how much our daughters need us to be women who were once young, once daughters, and once girls, we give them a new hope for staying whole if they decide to venture into motherhood themselves.

You can rest assured that when we choose to improve our daughter's relationship with food and body, we're doing challenging, vital work. By using the IFM to strengthen our daughter's eating competence, we're also reaching back into ourselves and mending our own relationship with food, body, eating, and weight. If our mothers suffered, we may even be reaching further back and mending her relationship with these crucial parts of existence, too. When we are successful in our work even a little bit, we change the future for ourselves, our daughters, their daughters, and anyone else who is touched by the ways we eat, talk about food, move, and feel about our bodies. We protect our girls from wasting their brilliance or energy on something as distracting and damaging as dieting. We help them become more of themselves and, in that, they have so much more to offer the world.

If you feel so compelled, I invite you to help mend the soul of the women eaters of the world by taking this work one step further. Share your own stories, your struggles, your transformations, and your triumphs with other mothers. You can do this through writing or speaking, online or in person, with friends, partners, or strangers, to groups of thousands or singular individuals. The most important part is to not stay silent. Sharing all we've gone through with eating (and not eating) can help others fell less alone or ashamed, as well as give them a chance to see their own situation with new eyes.

And finally, if you're still teetering between the two worlds—to diet or not to diet, to worry about body shape and size or to put it to rest for good—please know that help is here for you. You can find professional support, articles, workshops, courses, and ways to connect with a community of like-minded mothers at NourishHer.com. All the resources are designed to help women redefine their relationships to food and body so that they can build happier, healthier lives for themselves and their children.

ACKNOWLEDGMENTS

I CAN HARDLY BELIEVE I MADE IT TO THE END MYSELF, BUT HERE we are. Thanks goes to you, dear reader, for your precious time and patience with the content of this book and for being so invested in helping a young woman in your life. I'm 100% certain the world needs more people like you.

I owe so much gratitude to my husband, an unsuspecting hero in my mission to bring the idea for this book to life. From the hundreds of moments you stood patiently in the kitchen listening to me question everything to the limitless hours you spent caring for, entertaining, and feeding our daughters to make space for all of my typing, thinking, researching, and dreaming, thank you. Without a doubt, this book would not exist without your quiet patience and love.

And hip, hip, hooray to my daughters, who seemed to understand the importance of what I was doing for so many hours "on the third floor" and never questioned why I always went to work in my pajamas. To say you're the inspiration for my deep need to finally mend my relationship with my body would be an understatement. Mothering you made me do it, most certainly.

A huge thanks also goes to my fellow AKIMBO groupies, Frauke and Tasha. If I've failed as an author before, it was because I didn't understand that writing is not a solitary act. Frauke, thank you for being the midwife to this project; for meeting me at the brink of my New York mornings, listening as I cried and whined, staying steady in the act of showing up to birth your own words beside me, and having the patience to move me along when I was most unsure. I'm so grateful to have a gentle, writerly soul across from me during my most vulnerable moments. And thank you, Tasha, for picking me out of the TCW crowd; when I started writing about my own relationship with food and my daughter, you took the time to tell me you heard me. Your encouragement pushed me to go deeper and turn this into a book about so much more than what I'd originally envisioned it could be. In moments when I feared telling the truth of the matter, I'd imagine I was speaking only to you—and I think, for the most part, it worked. Thank you for being willing to hear it all and for telling me your own courageous, raw, and unfiltered stories, my writer friend.

Thank you to my editor, Ariel Curry, who somehow knew the very best way to push me out of the hiding spot that is perfectionism was to quote Dolly Parton. You went above and beyond for me as a guide on this project and I'm so excited for the many other writers who will enjoy the blessing of working with you in the future.

A special thank you to Katja Rowell for the exceptional generosity and patience you showed me in taking the time to point out at least a few of my blind spots on this topic. If the anti-diet, weight-inclusive landscape was filled with as much kindness and understanding as you showed me, then we'd likely be able to pull an infinitely larger number of professionals into it. Thank you for being an unintentional mentor to me in more than one way.

It's important to note the fact that I'm the recipient of a lot of privilege. Without those unearned benefits, I likely would not have been able to write or publish this work. We need more stories about eating and not eating from more diverse experiences and from both sides of the counseling table. If you have one to tell and need help in amplifying your voice, please reach out to me at amelia@ameliasherry.com. If I can't help you, I will do whatever I can to connect you with someone who can.

Lastly, thank you to every patient or client who had the courage to be vulnerable with me in sharing your personal stories about eating, dieting, parenting, and being parented. Your honesty is what made me realize this book had to be written—and with any luck, your stories will help other young women receive deeper acceptance, connection, and understanding from their own mothers on these complex topics, too.

NOTES

WHY GIRLS?

1. Nagata, Jason M., Kyle T. Ganson, and Stuart B. Murray. "Eating Disorders in Adolescent Boys and Young Men: An Update." *Current Opinion in Pediatrics* 32, no. 4 (August 2020): 476–81. https://doi.org/10.1097/MOP.0000000000000911.

2. Hudson, James I., Eva Hiripi, Harrison G. Pope, and Ronald C. Kessler. "The Prevalence and Correlates of Eating Disorders in the National Comorbidity Survey Replication." *Biological Psychiatry* 61, no. 3 (February 2007): 348–58. https://doi.org/10.1016/j.biopsych.2006.03.040.

3. Yoon, Cynthia, Susan M. Mason, Laura Hooper, Marla E. Eisenberg, and Dianne Neumark-Sztainer. "Disordered Eating Behaviors and 15-Year Trajectories in Body Mass Index: Findings from Project EAT." *The Journal of Adolescent Health: Official Publication of the Society for Adolescent Medicine* 66, no. 2 (February 2020): 181–88. https://doi.org/10.1016/j.jadohealth.2019.08.012.

4. Reba-Harrelson, L., A. Von Holle, R. M. Hamer, R. Swann, M. L. Reyes, and C. M. Bulik. "Patterns and Prevalence of Disordered Eating and Weight Control Behaviors in Women Ages 25-45." *Eating and Weight Disorders: EWD* 14, no. 4 (December 2009): e190-198. https://doi.org/10.1007/BF03325116.

5. Pennebaker, James W. "Expressive Writing in Psychological Science." *Perspectives on Psychological Science* 13, no. 2 (March 2018): 226–29. https://doi.org/10.1177/1745691617707315.

CHAPTER ONE: EATING WHILE FEMALE

1. Reba-Harrelson, L., A. Von Holle, R. M. Hamer, R. Swann, M. L. Reyes, and C. M. Bulik. "Patterns and Prevalence of Disordered Eating and Weight Control Behaviors in Women Ages 25–45." *Eating and Weight Disorders - Studies on Anorexia, Bulimia and Obesity* 14, no. 4 (December 2009): 190–98. https://doi.org/10.1007/BF03325116 .

2. Sarfan, Laurel D., Elise M. Clerkin, Bethany A. Teachman, and April R. Smith. "Do Thoughts about Dieting Matter? Testing the Relationship between Thoughts about Dieting, Body Shape Concerns, and State Self-Esteem." *Journal of Behavior Therapy and Experimental Psychiatry* 62 (March 2019): 7–14. https://doi.org/10.1016/j.jbtep.2018.08.005 .

3. "Body Mass Index (BMI) Measurement in Schools," August 10, 2022. https://www.cdc.gov/healthyschools/obesity/bmi/bmi_measurement_schools.htm.

4. Kurth, C. L., D. D. Krahn, K. Nairn, and A. Drewnowski. "The Severity of Dieting and Bingeing Behaviors in College Women: Interview Validation of Survey Data." *Journal of Psychiatric Research* 29, no. 3 (June 1995): 211–25. https://doi.org/10.1016/0022-3956(95)00002-m .

CHAPTER TWO: CREATING YOUR INTENTIONAL FEEDING MINDSET (IFM)

1. Ellyn Satter Institute. "Eating Competence Encourages Eating Wisely and Well." Accessed October 3, 2022. https://www.ellynsatterinstitute.org/satter-eating-competence-model/.

2. Krall, Jodi S, and Barbara Lohse. "Validation of a Measure of the Satter Eating Competence Model with Low-Income Females." *International Journal of Behavioral Nutrition and Physical Activity* 8, no. 1 (2011): 26. https://doi.org/10.1186/1479-5868-8-26; Lohse, Barbara, Ellyn Satter, Tanya Horacek, Tesfayi Gebreselassie, and Mary Jane Oakland. "Measuring Eating Competence: Psychometric Properties and Validity of the EcSatter Inventory." *Journal of Nutrition Education and Behavior* 39, no. 5 (September 2007): S154–66. https://doi.org/10.1016/j.jneb.2007.04.371 .

3. Godleski, Stephanie, Barbara Lohse, and Jodi S. Krall. 2019. "Satter Eating Competence Inventory Subscale Restructure after Confirmatory Factor Analysis." *Journal of Nutrition Education and Behavior* 51 (8): 1003–10. https://doi.org/10.1016/j.jneb.2019.05.287; Krall, et al. "Validation of a Measure of the Satter Eating Competence Model with Low-Income Females."; Lohse, Barbara, Kathryn Faulring, Diane C. Mitchell, and Leslie Cunningham-Sabo. 'A Definition of 'Regular Meals' Driven by Dietary Quality Supports a Pragmatic Schedule." *Nutrients* 12, no. 9 (September 1, 2020): 2667 https://doi.org/10.3390/nu12092667; Lohse, Barbara, Melissa Pflugh Prescott, and Leslie Cunningham-Sabo. "Eating Competent Parents of 4th Grade Youth from a Predominantly Non-Hispanic White Sample Demonstrate More Healthful Eating Behaviors than Non-Eating Competent Parents." *Nutrients* 11, no. 7 (June 30, 2019): 1501. https://doi.org/10.3390/nu11071501; Greene, Geoffrey W., Susan M. Schembre, Adrienne A. White, Sharon L. Hoerr, Barbara Lohse, Suzanne Shoff, Tanya Horacek, et al. "Identifying Clusters of College Students at Elevated Health Risk Based on Eating and Exercise Behaviors and Psychosocial Determinants of Body Weight." *Journal of the American Dietetic Association* 111, no. 3 (March 2011): 394–400. https://doi.org/10.1016/j. jada.2010.11.011; Lohse, et al., "Measuring Eating Competence: Psychometric Properties and Validity of the EcSatter Inventory."; Lohse, Barbara, Regan L. Bailey, Jodi Stotts Krall, Denise E. Wall, and Diane C. Mitchell. "Diet Quality Is Related to Eating Competence in Cross-Sectional Sample of Low-Income Females Surveyed in Pennsylvania." *Appetite* 58, no. 2 (April 2012): 645–50. https://doi.org/10.1016/j.appet.2011.11.022; Tylka, Tracy L., Ihuoma U. Eneli, Ashley M. Kroon Van Diest, and Julie C. Lumeng. "Which Adaptive Maternal Eating Behaviors Predict Child Feeding Practices? An Examination with Mothers of 2- to 5-Year-Old Children." *Eating Behaviors* 14, no. 1 (January 2013): 57–63. https://doi. org/10.1016/j.eatbeh.2012.10.014; Tilles-Tirkkonen, Tanja, Kirsikka Aittola, Reija Männikkö, Pilvikki Absetz, Marjukka Kolehmainen, Ursula Schwab, Jaana Lindström, Timo Lakka, Jussi Pihlajamäki, and Leila Karhunen. "Eating Competence Is Associated with Lower Prevalence of Obesity and Better Insulin Sensitivity in Finnish Adults with Increased Risk for Type 2 Diabetes: The StopDia Study." *Nutrients* 12, no. 1 (December 30, 2019): 104. https://doi.org/10.3390/nu12010104; Lohse, Barbara, and Leslie Cunningham-Sabo. "Eating Competence of Hispanic Parents Is Associated with Attitudes and Behaviors That May Mediate Fruit and Vegetable-Related Behaviors of 4th Grade Youth." *The Journal of Nutrition* 142, no. 10 (October 1, 2012): 1903–9. https://doi.org/10.3945/ jn.112.164269; Lohse, Barbara, Tricia Psota, Ramón Estruch, Itziar Zazpe,

José V. Sorli, Jordi Salas-Salvadò, Mercè Serra, et al. "Eating Competence of Elderly Spanish Adults Is Associated with a Healthy Diet and a Favorable Cardiovascular Disease Risk Profile." *The Journal of Nutrition* 140, no. 7 (July 1, 2010): 1322–27. https://doi.org/10.3945/jn.109.120188; Psota, Tricia L., Barbara Lohse, and Sheila G. West. "Associations between Eating Competence and Cardiovascular Disease Biomarkers." *Journal of Nutrition Education and Behavior* 39, no. 5 (September 2007): S171–78. https://doi.org/10.1016/j.jneb.2007.05.004; Tanja, Tilles-Tirkkonen, Nuutinen Outi, Suominen Sakari, Liukkonen Jarmo, Poutanen Kaisa, and Karhunen Leila. "Preliminary Finnish Measures of Eating Competence Suggest Association with Health-Promoting Eating Patterns and Related Psychobehavioral Factors in 10–17 Year Old Adolescents." *Nutrients* 7, no. 5 (May 21, 2015): 3828–46. https://doi.org/10.3390/nu7053828; Quick, Virginia, Carol Byrd-Bredbenner, Adrienne A. White, Onikia Brown, Sarah Colby, Suzanne Shoff, Barbara Lohse, Tanya Horacek, Tanda Kidd, and Geoffrey Greene. "Eat, Sleep, Work, Play: Associations of Weight Status and Health-Related Behaviors among Young Adult College Students." *American Journal of Health Promotion* 29, no. 2 (November 2014): e64–72. https://doi.org/10.4278/ajhp.130327-QUAN-130.

4. Satter, Ellyn. 2007. "Eating Competence: Nutrition Education with the Satter Eating Competence Model." *Journal of Nutrition Education and Behavior* 39 (5): S189–94. https://doi.org/10.1016/j.jneb.2007.04.177; Satter, Ellyn. 2007. "Eating Competence: Definition and Evidence for the Satter Eating Competence Model." *Journal of Nutrition Education and Behavior* 39 (5): S142–53. https://doi.org/10.1016/j.jneb.2007.01.006; Ellyn Satter, "Ellyn Satter's Treating the Dieting Casualty Vision Workshop Training Manual," (January 2020).

5. Lohse, Barbara, Ellyn Satter, and Kristen Arnold. 2014. "Development of a Tool to Assess Adherence to a Model of the Division of Responsibility in Feeding Young Children: Using Response Mapping to Capacitate Validation Measures." *Childhood Obesity* 10 (2): 153–68. https://doi.org/10.1089/chi.2013.0085;

6. Tylka et al., "Which Adaptive Maternal Eating Behaviors Predict Child Feeding Practices?"; Lohse et al., "Measuring Eating Competence."\\uc0\\u8220{}Measuring Eating Competence\\uc0\\u8221{}; Lohse, Satter, and Arnold, \\uc0\\u8220{}Development of a Tool to Assess Adherence to a Model of the Division of Responsibility in Feeding Young Children.\\uc0\\u8221{}","plainCitation":"Lohse, Satter, and Arnold, "Development of a Tool to Assess Adherence to a Model of the Division of Responsibility in Feeding Young Children"; Tylka et al., "Which Adaptive Maternal Eating

Behaviors Predict Child Feeding Practices?"; Lohse et al., "Measuring Eating Competence"; Lohse, Satter, and Arnold, "Development of a Tool to Assess Adherence to a Model of the Division of Responsibility in Feeding Young Children."","noteIndex":14},"citationItems":[{"id":4399,"uris":["ht tp://zotero.org/users/1707923/items/SJ96VZH7"],"itemData":{"id":4399 ,"type":"article-journal","abstract":"BACKGROUND: Accurate early assessment and targeted intervention with problematic parent/child feeding dynamics is critical for the prevention and treatment of child obesity. The division of responsibility in feeding (sDOR

CHAPTER THREE: INFLUENCE

1. Kelly, Amy M., Melanie Wall, Marla E. Eisenberg, Mary Story, and Dianne Neumark-Sztainer. "Adolescent Girls with High Body Satisfaction: Who Are They and What Can They Teach Us?" *Journal of Adolescent Health* 37, no. 5 (November 2005): 391–96. https://doi.org/10.1016/j.jadohealth.2004.08.008.

2. Gillison, Fiona B., Ava B. Lorenc, Ester F.C. Sleddens, Stefanie L. Williams, and Lou Atkinson. "Can It Be Harmful for Parents to Talk to Their Child about Their Weight? A Meta-Analysis." *Preventive Medicine* 93 (December 2016): 135–46. https://doi.org/10.1016/j.ypmed.2016.10.010.

3. Berge, Jerica M., Rich MacLehose, Katie A. Loth, Marla Eisenberg, Michaela M. Bucchianeri, and Dianne Neumark-Sztainer. "Parent Conversations About Healthful Eating and Weight: Associations With Adolescent Disordered Eating Behaviors." *JAMA Pediatrics* 167, no. 8 (August 1, 2013): 746. https://doi.org/10.1001/jamapediatrics.2013.78; Bauer, Katherine W, Michaela M Bucchianeri, and Dianne Neumark-Sztainer. "Mother-Reported Parental Weight Talk and Adolescent Girls' Emotional Health, Weight Control Attempts, and Disordered Eating Behaviors." *Journal of Eating Disorders* 1, no. 1 (December 2013): 45. https://doi.org/10.1186/2050-2974-1-45; Neumark-Sztainer, Dianne, Katherine W. Bauer, Sarah Friend, Peter J. Hannan, Mary Story, and Jerica M. Berge. "Family Weight Talk and Dieting: How Much Do They Matter for Body Dissatisfaction and Disordered Eating Behaviors in Adolescent Girls?" *Journal of Adolescent Health* 47, no. 3 (September 2010): 270–76. https://doi.org/10.1016/j.jadohealth.2010.02.001.793, mean age=14.4

4. Berge, Jerica M., Megan R. Winkler, Nicole Larson, Jonathan Miller, Ann F. Haynos, and Dianne Neumark-Sztainer. "Intergenerational Transmission

of Parent Encouragement to Diet From Adolescence Into Adulthood." *Pediatrics* 141, no. 4 (April 1, 2018): e20172955. https://doi.org/10.1542/peds.2017-2955.

5. Klein, Kelly M., Tiffany A. Brown, Grace A. Kennedy, and Pamela K. Keel. "Examination of Parental Dieting and Comments as Risk Factors for Increased Drive for Thinness in Men and Women at 20-Year Follow-up: Examination of Parental Dieting." *International Journal of Eating Disorders* 50, no. 5 (May 2017): 490–97. https://doi.org/10.1002/eat.22599; Balantekin, Katherine N. "The Influence of Parental Dieting Behavior on Child Dieting Behavior and Weight Status." *Current Obesity Reports* 8, no. 2 (June 2019): 137–44. https://doi.org/10.1007/s13679-019-00338-0; Neumark-Sztainer et al., "Family Weight Talk and Dieting"; Puhl, Rebecca M., and Mary S. Himmelstein. "Weight Bias Internalization Among Adolescents Seeking Weight Loss: Implications for Eating Behaviors and Parental Communication." *Frontiers in Psychology* 9 (November 21, 2018): 2271. https://doi.org/10.3389/fpsyg.2018.02271; Berge, et al., "Parent Conversations About Healthful Eating and Weight: Associations With Adolescent Disordered Eating Behaviors."; Berge, Jerica M., Richard F. MacLehose, Katie A. Loth, Marla E. Eisenberg, Jayne A. Fulkerson, and Dianne Neumark-Sztainer. "Parent-Adolescent Conversations about Eating, Physical Activity and Weight: Prevalence across Sociodemographic Characteristics and Associations with Adolescent Weight and Weight-Related Behaviors." *Journal of Behavioral Medicine* 38, no. 1 (February 2015): 122–35. https://doi.org/10.1007/s10865-014-9584-3; Gillison, et. al, "Can It Be Harmful for Parents to Talk to Their Child about Their Weight? A Meta-Analysis."

6. Hillard, Erin E., Dawn M. Gondoli, Alexandra F. Corning, and Rebecca A. Morrissey. "In It Together: Mother Talk of Weight Concerns Moderates Negative Outcomes of Encouragement to Lose Weight on Daughter Body Dissatisfaction and Disordered Eating." *Body Image* 16 (March 2016): 21–27. https://doi.org/10.1016/j.bodyim.2015.09.004.7.

7. Abramovitz, Beth A, and Leann L Birch. "Five-Year-Old Girls' Ideas About Dieting Are Predicted by Their Mothers' Dieting." *Journal of the American Dietetic Association* 100, no. 10 (October 2000): 1157–63. https://doi.org/10.1016/S0002-8223(00)00339-4; Davison, Kirsten Krahnstoever, and Leann Lipps Birch. "Weight Status, Parent Reaction, and Self-Concept in Five-Year-Old Girls." *Pediatrics* 107, no. 1 (January 1, 2001): 46–53. https://doi.org/10.1542/peds.107.1.46; Davison, Kirsten Krahnstoever, Charlotte N. Markey, and Leann L. Birch. "A Longitudinal Examination of Patterns in Girls' Weight Concerns and Body Dissatisfaction from Ages 5 to 9 Years."

International Journal of Eating Disorders 33, no. 3 (April 2003): 320–32. https://doi.org/10.1002/eat.10142; McDow, Kendra B., Duong T. Nguyen, Kirsten A. Herrick, and Lara J. Akinbami. "Attempts to Lose Weight Among Adolescents Aged 15-19 in the United States, 2013-2016." *NCHS Data Brief*, no. 340 (July 2019): 1–8; "Eating Disorders: About More Than Just Food." National Institute of Mental Health: Office of Science Policy, Planning, and Communications, Revise 2021. https://www.nimh.nih.gov/sites/default/files/documents/health/publications/eating-disorders/21-MH-4901-EatingDisorders_0.pdf;

8. "Fatphobia | Boston Medical Center." Accessed October 18, 2022. https://www.bmc.org/glossary-culture-transformation/fatphobia.

9. Puhl, Rebecca, and Young Suh. "Health Consequences of Weight Stigma: Implications for Obesity Prevention and Treatment." *Current Obesity Reports* 4, no. 2 (June 2015): 182–90. https://doi.org/10.1007/s13679-015-0153-z.

10. Puhl, Rebecca M., and Mary S. Himmelstein. 2018. "Weight Bias Internalization among Adolescents Seeking Weight Loss: Implications for Eating Behaviors and Parental Communication." *Frontiers in Psychology* 9 (November). https://doi.org/10.3389/fpsyg.2018.02271.

11. Pont, Stephen J., Rebecca Puhl, Stephen R. Cook, and Wendelin Slusser. 2017. "Stigma Experienced by Children and Adolescents with Obesity." *Pediatrics* 140 (6): e20173034. https://doi.org/10.1542/peds.2017-3034.

12. Spiel, Emma C., Susan J. Paxton, and Zali Yager. "Weight Attitudes in 3- to 5-Year-Old Children: Age Differences and Cross-Sectional Predictors." *Body Image* 9, no. 4 (September 2012): 524–27. https://doi.org/10.1016/j.bodyim.2012.07.006; Su, Wei, and Di Santo Aurelia. "Preschool Children's Perceptions of Overweight Peers." *Journal of Early Childhood Research* 10, no. 1 (February 2012): 19–31. https://doi.org/10.1177/1476718X11407411.

13. Christensen, Vibeke T. "Does Parental Capital Influence the Prevalence of Child Overweight and Parental Perceptions of Child Weight-Level?" *Social Science & Medicine* 72, no. 4 (February 2011): 469–77. https://doi.org/10.1016/j.socscimed.2010.11.037; Aljunaibi, Abdulla, Abdishakur Abdulle, and Nico Nagelkerke. "Parental Weight Perceptions: A Cause for Concern in the Prevention and Management of Childhood Obesity in the United Arab Emirates." Edited by C. Mary Schooling. *PLoS ONE* 8, no. 3 (March 26, 2013): e59923. https://doi.org/10.1371/journal.pone.0059923; Robinson, Eric, and Angelina R. Sutin. "Parental Perception of Weight Status and Weight Gain Across Childhood." *Pediatrics* 137, no. 5 (May 1, 2016): e20153957. https://doi.org/10.1542/peds.2015-3957.

14. Germic, Eloise R., Stine Eckert, and Fred Vultee. "The Impact of Instagram Mommy Blogger Content on the Perceived Self-Efficacy of Mothers." *Social Media + Society* 7, no. 3 (July 2021): 205630512110416. https://doi.org/10.1177/20563051211041649; Ouvrein, Gaëlle. "Mommy Influencers: Helpful or Harmful? The Relationship between Exposure to Mommy Influencers and Perceived Parental Self-Efficacy among Mothers and Primigravida." *New Media & Society*, April 4, 2022, 146144482210862. https://doi.org/10.1177/14614448221086296; Song, Felicia Wu. "The Serious Business of Mommy Bloggers." *Contexts* 15, no. 3 (August 2016): 42–49. https://doi.org/10.1177/1536504216662234.

CHAPTER FOUR: WELL-BEING

1. "Constitution of the World Health Organization." Accessed October 18, 2022. https://www.who.int/about/governance/constitution.

2. Field, Alison E., S. B. Austin, C. B. Taylor, Susan Malspeis, Bernard Rosner, Helaine R. Rockett, Matthew W. Gillman, and Graham A. Colditz. "Relation Between Dieting and Weight Change Among Preadolescents and Adolescents." *Pediatrics* 112, no. 4 (October 1, 2003): 900–906. https://doi.org/10.1542/peds.112.4.900.

3. Arroyo, Analisa, Chris Segrin, and Kristin K. Andersen. "Intergenerational Transmission of Disordered Eating: Direct and Indirect Maternal Communication among Grandmothers, Mothers, and Daughters." *Body Image* 20 (March 2017): 107–15. https://doi.org/10.1016/j.bodyim.2017.01.001; Berge et al., "Parent Conversations about Healthful Eating and Weight"; Berge et al., "Parent-Adolescent Conversations about Eating, Physical Activity and Weight"; Berge et al., "Intergenerational Transmission of Parent Encouragement to Diet From Adolescence Into Adulthood."dieting, bulimia and food preoccupation, and oral control

4. Montmayeur, Jean-Pierre, and Johannes Le Coutre. "Chapter 8: Neural Representation of Fat Texture in the Mouth." Essay. In *Fat Detection Taste, Texture, and Post Ingestive Effects*. Boca Raton, FL: CRC Press/Taylor & Francis, 2010. https://pubmed.ncbi.nlm.nih.gov/21452476/; Li, Mengtong, Hwei-Ee Tan, Zhengyuan Lu, Katherine S. Tsang, Ashley J. Chung, and Charles S. Zuker. "Gut–Brain Circuits for Fat Preference." *Nature*, September 7, 2022, 1–9. https://doi.org/10.1038/s41586-022-05266-z.

5. Baikie, Karen A., and Kay Wilhelm. "Emotional and Physical Health Benefits of Expressive Writing." *Advances in Psychiatric Treatment* 11, no. 5 (September 2005): 338–46. https://doi.org/10.1192/apt.11.5.338.

6. Strien, Tatjana van, Harriëtte M. Snoek, Carmen S. van der Zwaluw, and Rutger C.M.E. Engels. "Parental Control and the Dopamine D2 Receptor Gene (DRD2) Interaction on Emotional Eating in Adolescence." *Appetite* 54, no. 2 (April 2010): 255–61. https://doi.org/10.1016/j.appet.2009.11.006; Strien, Tatjana van, Carmen S. van der Zwaluw, and Rutger C.M.E. Engels. "Emotional Eating in Adolescents: A Gene (SLC6A4/5-HTT) – Depressive Feelings Interaction Analysis." *Journal of Psychiatric Research* 44, no. 15 (November 2010): 1035–42. https://doi.org/10.1016/j.jpsychires.2010.03.012.

7. Lieberman, Matthew D., Naomi I. Eisenberger, Molly J. Crockett, Sabrina M. Tom, Jennifer H. Pfeifer, and Baldwin M. Way. "Putting Feelings Into Words." *Psychological Science* 18, no. 5 (May 2007): 421–28. https://doi.org/10.1111/j.1467-9280.2007.01916.x; Siegel, Daniel J., and Tina Payne Bryson. *The Whole-Brain Child: 12 Revolutionary Strategies to Nurture Your Child's Developing Mind*. Vancouver, B.C.: Langara College, 2016.

8. Woolley, Kaitlin, and Ayelet Fishbach. 2019. "Shared Plates, Shared Minds: Consuming from a Shared Plate Promotes Cooperation." *Psychological Science* 30 (4): 541–52. https://doi.org/10.1177/0956797619830633; Cao, Jiyin, Dejun Tony Kong, and Adam D. Galinsky. 2020. "Breaking Bread Produces Bigger Pies: An Empirical Extension of Shared Eating to Negotiations and a Commentary on Woolley and Fishbach (2019)." *Psychological Science* 31 (10): 1340–45. https://doi.org/10.1177/0956797620939532.

9. Berge, Jerica M., Vivienne M. Hazzard, Nicole Larson, Samantha L. Hahn, Rebecca L. Emery, and Dianne Neumark-Sztainer. "Are There Protective Associations between Family/Shared Meal Routines during COVID-19 and Dietary Health and Emotional Well-Being in Diverse Young Adults?" *Preventive Medicine Reports* 24 (September 28, 2021): 101575. https://doi.org/10.1016/j.pmedr.2021.101575; Fulkerson, Jayne A., Mary Story, Alison Mellin, Nancy Leffert, Dianne Neumark-Sztainer, Simone French. "Family Dinner Meal Frequency and Adolescent Development: Relationships with Developmental Assets and High-Risk Behaviors." *Journal of Adolescent Health* 39, no. 3 (September 1, 2006): 337–45. https://doi.org/10.1016/j.jadohealth.2005.12.026; Fulkerson, Jayne A., Martha Y. Kubik, Mary Story, Leslie Lytle, and Chrisa Arcan. 2009. "Are There Nutritional and Other Benefits Associated with Family Meals among At-Risk Youth?" *Journal of Adolescent Health* 45 (4): 389–95. https://doi.org/10.1016/j.jado-

health.2009.02.011; Fulkerson, Jayne A., Sarah Friend, Melissa Horning, Colleen Flattum, Michelle Draxten, Dianne Neumark-Sztainer, Olga Gurvich, Ann Garwick, Mary Story, and Martha Y. Kubik. 2018. "Family Home Food Environment and Nutrition-Related Parent and Child Personal and Behavioral Outcomes of the Healthy Home Offerings via the Mealtime Environment (HOME) plus Program: A Randomized Controlled Trial." *Journal of the Academy of Nutrition and Dietetics* 118 (2): 240–51. https://doi. org/10.1016/j.jand.2017.04.006; Horning, Melissa L., Jayne A. Fulkerson, Sarah E. Friend, and Dianne Neumark-Sztainer. 2016. "Associations among Nine Family Dinner Frequency Measures and Child Weight, Dietary, and Psychosocial Outcomes." *Journal of the Academy of Nutrition and Dietetics* 116 (6): 991–99. https://doi.org/10.1016/j.jand.2015.12.018; Robson, Shannon M., Mary Beth McCullough, Samantha Rex, Marcus R. Munafò, and Gemma Taylor. 2020. "Family Meal Frequency, Diet, and Family Functioning: A Systematic Review with Meta-Analyses." *Journal of Nutrition Education and Behavior* 52 (5): 553–64. https://doi.org/10.1016/j. jneb.2019.12.012; Utter, Jennifer, Nicole Larson, Jerica M. Berge, Marla E. Eisenberg, Jayne A. Fulkerson, and Dianne Neumark-Sztainer. 2018. "Family Meals among Parents: Associations with Nutritional, Social and Emotional Wellbeing." *Preventive Medicine* 113 (August): 7–12. https://doi. org/10.1016/j.ypmed.2018.05.006; Utter, Jennifer, Simon Denny, Elizabeth Robinson, Theresa Fleming, Shanthi Ameratunga, and Sue Grant. 2013. "Family Meals and the Well-Being of Adolescents." *Journal of Paediatrics and Child Health* 49 (11): 906–11. https://doi.org/10.1111/jpc.12428.

10. Elgar, Frank J., Anthony Napoletano, Grace Saul, Melanie A. Dirks, Wendy Craig, V. Paul Poteat, Melissa Holt, and Brian W. Koenig. 2014. "Cyberbullying Victimization and Mental Health in Adolescents and the Moderating Role of Family Dinners." *JAMA Pediatrics* 168 (11): 1015. https://doi.org/10.1001/jamapediatrics.2014.1223.

11. Chae, Wonjeong, Yeong Jun Ju, Jaeyong Shin, Sung-In Jang, and Eun-Cheol Park. 2018. "Association between Eating Behaviour and Diet Quality: Eating Alone vs. Eating with Others." *Nutrition Journal* 17 (1). https://doi. org/10.1186/s12937-018-0424-0; Conklin, Annalijn I., Nita G. Forouhi, Paul Surtees, Kay-Tee Khaw, Nicholas J. Wareham, and Pablo Monsivais. 2014. "Social Relationships and Healthful Dietary Behaviour: Evidence from Over-50s in the EPIC Cohort, UK." *Social Science & Medicine* 100 (January): 167–75. https://doi.org/10.1016/j.socscimed.2013.08.018.

12. Dunbar, R. I. M. 2017. "Breaking Bread: The Functions of Social Eating." *Adaptive Human Behavior and Physiology* 3 (3): 198–211. https://doi. org/10.1007/s40750-017-0061-4.

CHAPTER FIVE: WEIGHT

1. Flegal, Katherine M., Brian K. Kit, Heather Orpana, and Barry I. Graubard. 2013. "Association of All-Cause Mortality with Overweight and Obesity Using Standard Body Mass Index Categories." *JAMA* 309 (1): 71. https://doi.org/10.1001/jama 2012.113905.

2. Wright, Charlotte M, Louise Parker, Douglas Lamont, and Alan W Craft. 2001. "Implications of Childhood Obesity for Adult Health: Findings from Thousand Families Cohort Study." *BMJ : British Medical Journal* 323 (7324): 1280–84. https://www.ncbi.nlm.nih.gov/pmc/articles/PMC60301/.

3. Freedman, D. S., L. K. Khan, W. H. Dietz, S. R. Srinivasan, and G. S. Berenson. 2001. "Relationship of Childhood Obesity to Coronary Heart Disease Risk Factors in Adulthood: The Bogalusa Heart Study." *PEDIATRICS* 108 (3): 712–18. https://doi.org/10.1542/peds.108.3.712; Lloyd, L J, S C Langley-Evans, and S McMullen. 2011. "Childhood Obesity and Risk of the Adult Metabolic Syndrome: A Systematic Review." *International Journal of Obesity* 36 (1): 1–11. https://doi.org/10.1038/ijo.2011.186; Wright et al., "Implications of Childhood Obesity for Adult Health: Findings from Thousand Families Cohort Study."

4. Cole, T. J. 2000. "Establishing a Standard Definition for Child Overweight and Obesity Worldwide: International Survey." *BMJ* 320 (7244): 1240–40. https://doi.org/10.1136/bmj.320.7244.1240.

5. Wang, Zhiqiang, Meina Liu, Tania Pan, and Shilu Tong. 2016. "Lower Mortality Associated with Overweight in the U.S. National Health Interview Survey." *Medicine* 95 (2): e2424. https://doi.org/10.1097/md.0000000000002424; McGee, Daniel L. 2005. "Body Mass Index and Mortality: A Meta-Analysis Based on Person-Level Data from Twenty-Six Observational Studies." *Annals of Epidemiology* 15 (2): 87–97. https://doi.org/10.1016/j.annepidem.2004.05.012; Flegal et al., "Association of All-Cause Mortality With Overweight and Obesity Using Standard Body Mass Index Categories"; Flegal, Katherine M. 2005. "Excess Deaths Associated with Underweight, Overweight, and Obesity." *JAMA* 293 (15): 1861. https://doi.org/10.1001/jama.293.15.1861; Jerant, Anthony, and Peter Franks. 2012. "Body Mass Index, Diabetes, Hypertension, and Short-Term Mortality: A Population-Based Observational Study, 2000-2006." *Journal of the American Board of Family Medicine: JABFM* 25 (4): 422–31. https://doi.org/10.3122/jabfm.2012.04.110289.

6. Bacon, Linda, and Lucy Aphramor. 2011. "Weight Science: Evaluating the Evidence for a Paradigm Shift." *Nutrition Journal* 10 (1). https://doi.org/10.1186/1475-2891-10-9.

7. Sim, L. A., J. Lebow, and M. Billings. 2013. "Eating Disorders in Adolescents with a History of Obesity." *PEDIATRICS* 132 (4): e1026–30. https://doi.org/10.1542/peds.2012-3940.

8. Golden, N. H., M. Schneider, and C. Wood. 2016. "Preventing Obesity and Eating Disorders in Adolescents." *PEDIATRICS* 138 (3): e20161649–49. https://doi.org/10.1542/peds.2016-1649.

9. Mcgonigal, Kelly. 2019. *The Joy of Movement: How Exercise Helps Us Find Happiness, Hope, Connection, and Courage.* New York: Avery; Kramer, Eydie. 2019. "2.2 Physiological Benefits." Open.lib.umn.edu. 2019. https://open.lib.umn.edu/physicalactivity/chapter/2-2-physiological-benefits/.

10. Spiegel, Karine, Esra Tasali, Rachel Leproult, and Eve Van Cauter. 2009. "Effects of Poor and Short Sleep on Glucose Metabolism and Obesity Risk." *Nature Reviews Endocrinology* 5 (5): 253–61. https://doi.org/10.1038/nrendo.2009.23; Besedovsky, Luciana, Tanja Lange, and Jan Born. 2011. "Sleep and Immune Function." *Pflügers Archiv - European Journal of Physiology* 463 (1): 121–37. https://doi.org/10.1007/s00424-011-1044-0; Greer, Stephanie M., Andrea N. Goldstein, and Matthew P. Walker. 2013. "The Impact of Sleep Deprivation on Food Desire in the Human Brain." *Nature Communications* 4 (1). https://doi.org/10.1038/ncomms3259; Kim, Tae Won, Jong-Hyun Jeong, and Seung-Chul Hong. 2015. "The Impact of Sleep and Circadian Disturbance on Hormones and Metabolism." *International Journal of Endocrinology* 2015: 1–9. https://doi.org/10.1155/2015/591729; Scott, Alexander J, Thomas L Webb, and Georgina Rowse. 2017. "Does Improving Sleep Lead to Better Mental Health? A Protocol for a Meta-Analytic Review of Randomised Controlled Trials." *BMJ Open* 7 (9): e016873. https://doi.org/10.1136/bmjopen-2017-016873; Cousins, James N., Karen Sasmita, and Michael W. L. Chee. 2017. "Memory Encoding Is Impaired after Multiple Nights of Partial Sleep Restriction." *Journal of Sleep Research* 27 (1): 138–45. https://doi.org/10.1111/jsr.12578.

11. Yaribeygi, Habib, Yunes Panahi, Hedayat Sahraei, Thomas P Johnston, and Amirhossein Sahebkar. 2017. "The Impact of Stress on Body Function: A Review." *EXCLI Journal* 16 (1): 1057–72. https://doi.org/10.17179/excli2017-480.

12. Satter, Ellyn. 2000. *Child of Mine: Feeding with Love and Good Sense.* Palo Alto, Calif.: Bull Pub.; Berkeley, Ca. (34)

CHAPTER SIX: TRUST

1. Satter, Ellyn. 2011. *Secrets of Feeding a Healthy Family: How to Eat, How to Raise Good Eaters, How to Cook.* New York: Kelcy Press. "Appendix I Children and Food Regulation." (263).

2. Hahn-Holbrook, Jennifer, Darby Saxbe, Christine Bixby, Caroline Steele, and Laura Glynn. 2019. "Human Milk as 'Chrononutrition': Implications for Child Health and Development." *Pediatric Research* 85 (7): 936–42. https://doi.org/10.1038/s41390-019-0368-x; Czosnykowska-Łukacka, Matylda, Barbara Królak-Olejnik, and Magdalena Orczyk-Pawiłowicz. 2018. "Breast Milk Macronutrient Components in Prolonged Lactation." *Nutrients* 10 (12): 1893. https://doi.org/10.3390/nu10121893.

3. Haycraft, Emma, Huw Goodwin, and Caroline Meyer. 2014. "Adolescents' Level of Eating Psychopathology Is Related to Perceptions of Their Parents' Current Feeding Practices." *Journal of Adolescent Health* 54 (2): 204–8. https://doi.org/10.1016/j.jadohealth.2013.08.007.

4. Ellis, Jordan M., Amy T. Galloway, Rose Mary Webb, Denise M. Martz, and Claire V. Farrow. 2016. "Recollections of Pressure to Eat during Childhood, but Not Picky Eating, Predict Young Adult Eating Behavior." *Appetite* 97 (February): 58–63. https://doi.org/10.1016/j.appet.2015.11.020.

5. Orrell-Valente, Joan K., Laura G. Hill, Whitney A. Brechwald, Kenneth A. Dodge, Gregory S. Pettit, and John E. Bates. "'Just Three More Bites': An Observational Analysis of Parents' Socialization of Children's Eating at Mealtime." *Appetite* 48, no. 1 (January 2007): 37–45. https://doi.org/10.1016/j.appet.2006.06.006.

6. Lilenfeld, Lisa R., Walter H. Kaye, Catherine G. Greeno, Kathleen R. Merikangas, Katherine Plotnicov, Christine Pollice, Radhika Rao, Michael Strober, Cynthia M. Bulik, and Linda Nagy. 1998. "A Controlled Family Study of Anorexia Nervosa and Bulimia Nervosa." *Archives of General Psychiatry* 55 (7): 603 https://doi.org/10.1001/archpsyc.55.7.603; Strober, M. 2000. "Controlled Family Study of Anorexia Nervosa and Bulimia Nervosa: Evidence of Shared Liability and Transmission of Partial Syndromes." *American Journal of Psychiatry* 157 (3): 393–401. https://doi.org/10.1176/appi.ajp.157.3.393; Pike, K. M., and J. Rodin. 1991. "Mothers, Daughters, and Disordered Eating." *Journal of Abnormal Psychology* 100 (2): 198–204. https://doi.org/10.1037//0021-843x.100.2.198.

7. Hood, MY, LL Moore, A Sundarajan-Ramamurti, M Singer, LA Cupples, and RC Ellison. 2000. "Parental Eating Attitudes and the Development of Obesity in Children. The Framingham Children's Study." *International Journal of Obesity* 24 (10): 1319–25. https://doi.org/10.1038/sj.ijo.0801396.

8. Gagnon-Girouard, M.-P., N. Carbonneau, M. Gendron, Y. Lussier, and C. Bégin. 2020. "Like Mother, like Daughter: Association of Maternal Negative Attitudes towards People of Higher Weight with Adult Daughters' Weight Bias." *Body Image* 34 (September): 277–81. https://doi.org/10.1016/j.bodyim.2020.07.004.

9. Baker, Jessica H., Hermine H. Maes, Lauren Lissner, Steven H. Aggen, Paul Lichtenstein, and Kenneth S. Kendler. 2009. "Genetic Risk Factors for Disordered Eating in Adolescent Males and Females." *Journal of Abnormal Psychology* 118 (3): 576–86. https://doi.org/10.1037/a0016314; Kaye, Walter H., Bernie Devlin, Nicole Barbarich, Cynthia M. Bulik, Laura Thornton, Silviu-Alin Bacanu, Manfred M. Fichter, et al. 2004. "Genetic Analysis of Bulimia Nervosa: Methods and Sample Description." *International Journal of Eating Disorders* 35 (4): 556–70. https://doi.org/10.1002/eat.10271.

10. Francis, Lori A., and Leann L. Birch. "Maternal Influences on Daughters' Restrained Eating Behavior." *Health Psychology : Official Journal of the Division of Health Psychology, American Psychological Association* 24, no. 6 (November 2005): 548–54. https://doi.org/10.1037/0278-6133.24.6.548

11. Haycraft, Emma, Huw Goodwin, and Caroline Meyer. "Adolescents' Level of Eating Psychopathology Is Related to Perceptions of Their Parents' Current Feeding Practices." *The Journal of Adolescent Health: Official Publication of the Society for Adolescent Medicine* 54, no. 2 (February 2014): 204–8. https://doi.org/10.1016/j.jadohealth.2013.08.007.

12. Ogden, Jane, and Jo Steward. "The Role of the Mother-Daughter Relationship in Explaining Weight Concern." *International Journal of Eating Disorders* 28, no. 1 (July 2000): 78–83. https://doi.org/10.1002/(SICI)1098-108X(200007)28:1<78::AID-EAT9>3.0.CO;2-N ; Cooper, Peter J., Elizabeth Whelan, Matthew Woolgar, Julian Morrell, and Lynne Murray. "Association between Childhood Feeding Problems and Maternal Eating Disorder: Role of the Family Environment." *The British Journal of Psychiatry* 184, no. 3 (March 2004): 210–15. https://doi.org/10.1192/bjp.184.3.210.

13. "Raise a Healthy Child Who Is a Joy to Feed." n.d. Ellyn Satter Institute. https://esiinstitute.wpengine.com/satter-feeding-dynamics-model/; Ellyn Satter Institute. "Raise a Healthy Child Who Is a Joy to Feed." Accessed October 3, 2022. https://www.ellynsatterinstitute.org/how-to-feed/.

14. Ellyn Satter, "Nutrition Education for Parents," (Feeding Dynamics or fdSatter) Treating the Dieting Casualty Vision Workshop Manual. (January 2020): (75); "Raise a Healthy Child Who Is a Joy to Feed." 2016. Ellyn Satter Institute. 2016. https://www.ellynsatterinstitute.org/satter-feeding-dynamics-model/.

CHAPTER SEVEN: ACCEPTANCE

1. Mendo-Lázaro, Santiago, Benito León-del-Barco, María-Isabel Polo-del-Río, Rocío Yuste-Tosina, and Víctor-María López-Ramos. "The Role of Parental Acceptance–Rejection in Emotional Instability During Adolescence." International Journal of Environmental Research and Public Health 16, no. 7 (April 2019): 1194. https://doi.org/10.3390/ijerph16071194 ; Dwairy, Marwan. "Parental Acceptance–Rejection: A Fourth Cross-Cultural Research on Parenting and Psychological Adjustment of Children." Journal of Child and Family Studies 19, no. 1 (February 1, 2010): 30–35. https://doi.org/10.1007/s10826-009-9338-y ; https://www.ncbi.nlm.nih.gov/pmc/articles/PMC7460297/

2. Ellyn Satter Institute. "Raise a Healthy Child Who Is a Joy to Feed." Accessed October 3, 2022. https://www.ellynsatterinstitute.org/how-to-feed/the-division-of-responsibility-in-feeding/; © Copyright 2022 by Ellyn Satter published at EllynSatterInstitute.org.

3. Mendo-Lázaro, et al., "The Role of Parental Acceptance–Rejection in Emotional Instability During Adolescence."

4. Berge, Jerica M., Caroline Hoppmann, Carrie Hanson, and Dianne Neumark-Sztainer. "Perspectives about Family Meals from Single-Headed and Dual-Headed Households: A Qualitative Analysis - PMC." PubMed Central (PMC). Accessed October 21, 2022. https://www.ncbi.nlm.nih.gov/pmc/articles/PMC3871516/.

CHAPTER EIGHT: SIMPLIFYING NUTRITION

1. Loth, Katie A., Richard F. MacLehose, Jayne A. Fulkerson, Scott Crow, and Dianne Neumark-Sztainer. "Are Food Restriction and Pressure-to-Eat Parenting Practices Associated with Adolescent Disordered Eating Behaviors?" The International Journal of Eating Disorders 47,

no. 3 (April 2014): 310–14. https://doi.org/10.1002/eat.22189; Polivy, Janet. "Psychological Consequences of Food Restriction." Journal of the American Dietetic Association 96, no. 6 (June 1, 1996): 589–92. https://doi.org/10.1016/S0002-8223(96)00161-7; Polivy, Janet, C. Peter Herman, and Jennifer S. Mills. "What Is Restrained Eating and How Do We Identify It?" Appetite 155 (December 1, 2020): 104820. https://doi.org/10.1016/j.appet.2020.104820.

CHAPTER NINE: MOVEMENT

1. Herring, Matthew P., Mats Hallgren, and Mark J. Campbell. 2017. "Acute Exercise Effects on Worry, State Anxiety, and Feelings of Energy and Fatigue among Young Women with Probable Generalized Anxiety Disorder: A Pilot Study." *Psychology of Sport and Exercise* 33 (November): 31–36. https://doi.org/10.1016/j.psychsport.2017.07.009; Herring, Matthew P., Derek Cl, Monroe, Brett R. Gordon, Mats Hallgren, and Mark J. Campbell. 2019. "Acute Exercise Effects among Young Adults with Analogue Generalized Anxiety Disorder." *Medicine & Science in Sports & Exercise* 51 (5): 962–69. https://doi.org/10.1249/mss.0000000000001860; Brand, Serge, Flora Colledge, Sebastian Ludyga, Raphael Emmenegger, Nadeem Kalak, Dena Sadeghi Bahmani, Edith Holsboer-Trachsler, Uwe Pühse, and Markus Gerber. 2018. "Acute Bouts of Exercising Improved Mood, Rumination and Social Interaction in Inpatients with Mental Disorders." *Frontiers in Psychology* 9 (March). https://doi.org/10.3389/fpsyg.2018.00249; Peluso, Marco Aurélio Monteiro, and Laura Helena Silveira Guerra de Andrade. 2005. "Physical Activity and Mental Health: The Association between Exercise and Mood." *Clinics* 60 (1): 61–70. https://doi.org/10.1590/s1807-59322005000100012; Norris, Richard, Douglas Carroll, and Raymond Cochrane. 1992. "The Effects of Physical Activity and Exercise Training on Psychological Stress and Well-Being in an Adolescent Population." *Journal of Psychosomatic Research* 36 (1): 55–65. https://doi.org/10.1016/0022-3999(92)90114-h.

2. Lang, Christin, Nadeem Kalak, Serge Brand, Edith Holsboer-Trachsler, Uwe Pühse, and Markus Gerber. 2016. "The Relationship between Physical Activity and Sleep from Mid Adolescence to Early Adulthood. A Systematic Review of Methodological Approaches and Meta-Analysis." *Sleep Medicine Reviews* 28 (August): 32–45. https://doi.org/10.1016/j.smrv.2015.07.004; Nixon, G M, J M D Thompson, D Y Han, D M O Becroft, P M Clark, E Robinson, K E Waldie, C J Wild, P N Black, and E A Mitchell. 2009.

"Falling Asleep: The Determinants of Sleep Latency." *Archives of Disease in Childhood* 94 (9): 686–89. https://doi.org/10.1136/adc.2009.157453.

3. Costilla, Vanessa C., and Amy E. Foxx-Orenstein. 2014. "Constipation." *Clinics in Geriatric Medicine* 30 (1): 107–15. https://doi.org/10.1016/j.cger.2013.10.001; Hosseini-Asl, Mohammad Kazem, Erfan Taherifard, and Mohammad Reza Mousavi. 2021. "The Effect of a Short-Term Physical Activity after Meals on Gastrointestinal Symptoms in Individuals with Functional Abdominal Bloating: A Randomized Clinical Trial." *Gastroenterology and Hepatology from Bed to Bench* 14 (1): 59–66. https://www.ncbi.nlm.nih.gov/pmc/articles/PMC8035544/.

4. Naugle, Kelly M., Roger B. Fillingim, and Joseph L. Riley. 2012. "A Meta-Analytic Review of the Hypoalgesic Effects of Exercise." *The Journal of Pain* 13 (12): 1139–50. https://doi.org/10.1016/j.jpain.2012.09.006.

5. Colberg, S. R., R. J. Sigal, B. Fernhall, J. G. Regensteiner, B. J. Blissmer, R. R. Rubin, L. Chasan-Taber, A. L. Albright, and B. Braun. 2010. "Exercise and Type 2 Diabetes: The American College of Sports Medicine and the American Diabetes Association: Joint Position Statement Executive Summary." *Diabetes Care* 33 (12): 2692–96. https://doi.org/10.2337/dc10-1548; Wellman, Robert J., Marie-Pierre Sylvestre, Patrick Abi Nader, Arnaud Chiolero, Miceline Mesidor, Erika N. Dugas, Gauthier Tougri, and Jennifer O'Loughlin. 2020. 'Intensity and Frequency of Physical Activity and High Blood Pressure in Adolescents: A Longitudinal Study." *The Journal of Clinical Hypertension* 22 (2): 283–90. https://doi.org/10.1111/jch.13806; Nieman, David C., and Laurel M. Wentz. 2019. "The Compelling Link between Physical Activity and the Body's Defense System." *Journal of Sport and Health Science* 8 (3): 201–17. https://doi.org/10.1016/j.jshs.2018.09.009.

6. Bidzan-Bluma, Ilona, and Małgorzata Lipowska. 2018. "Physical Activity and Cognitive Functioning of Children: A Systematic Review." *International Journal of Environmental Research and Public Health* 15 (4): 800. https://doi.org/10.3390/ijerph15040800; Hogan, Candice L., Jutta Mata, and Laura L. Carstensen. 2013. "Exercise Holds Immediate Benefits for Affect and Cognition in Younger and Older Adults." *Psychology and Aging* 28 (2): 587–94. https://doi.org/10.1037/a0032634.

7. Ratey, John J, and Eric Hagerman. 2008. *Spark: The Revolutionary New Science of Exercise and the Brain*. New York: Little, Brown.

8. Fernández-Bustos, Juan Gregorio, Álvaro Infantes-Paniagua, Ricardo Cuevas, and Onofre Ricardo Contreras. 2019. "Effect of Physical Activity on Self-Concept: Theoretical Model on the Mediation of Body Image

and Physical Self-Concept in Adolescents." *Frontiers in Psychology* 10 (July). https://doi.org/10.3389/fpsyg.2019.01537. ; Willow, Jason P. 2005. "Physical Activity Participation, Physical Self-Perceptions and Social Self-Esteem." *Medicine & Science in Sports & Exercise* 37 (Supplement): S371. https://doi.org/10.1249/00005768-200505001-01930.

9. Wallman-Jones, Amie, Pandelis Perakakis, Manos Tsakiris, and Mirko Schmidt. 2021. "Physical Activity and Interoceptive Processing: Theoretical Considerations for Future Research." *International Journal of Psychophysiology* 166 (August): 38–49. https://doi.org/10.1016/j.ijpsycho.2021.05.002.

10. Davis, Arran, Jacob Taylor, and Emma Cohen. 2015. "Social Bonds and Exercise: Evidence for a Reciprocal Relationship." Edited by Alex Mesoudi. *PLOS ONE* 10 (8): e0136705. https://doi.org/10.1371/journal. pone.0136705; Mcgonigal, Kelly. 2021. *The Joy of Movement: How Exercise Helps Us Find Happiness, Hope, Connection, and Courage.* S.L.: Avery Pub Group (34-35); Tarr, Bronwyn, Jacques Launay, Emma Cohen, and Robin Dunbar. 2015. "Synchrony and Exertion during Dance Independently Raise Pain Threshold and Encourage Social Bonding." *Biology Letters* 11 (10): 20150767. https://doi.org/10.1098/rsbl.2015.0767; Reddish, Paul, Eddie M. W. Tong, Jonathan Jong, Jonathan A. Lanman, and Harvey Whitehouse. 2016. "Collective Synchrony Increases Prosociality towards Non-Performers and Outgroup Members." *British Journal of Social Psychology* 55 (4): 722–38. https://doi.org/10.1111/bjso.12165..

11. Faith, Myles S., Mary Ann Leone, Tim S. Ayers, Moonseong Heo, and Angelo Pietrobelli. "Weight Criticism during Physical Activity, Coping Skills, and Reported Physical Activity in Children." Pediatrics 110, no. 2 Pt 1 (August 2002): e23. https://doi.org/10.1542/peds.110.2.e23; Davison, Kirsten Krahnstoever, and Glenn D. Deane. 2010. "The Consequence of Encouraging Girls to Be Active for Weight Loss." *Social Science & Medicine* 70 (4): 518–25. https://doi.org/10.1016/j.socscimed.2009.10.061.

12. Klesges, R. C., M. L. Shelton, and L. M. Klesges. "Effects of Television on Metabolic Rate: Potential Implications for Childhood Obesity." Pediatrics 91, no. 2 (February 1993): 281–86.

13. Pedersen, Jesper, Martin Gillies Banke Rasmussen, Sarah Overgaard Sørensen, Sofie Rath Mortensen, Line Grønholt Olesen, Jan Christian Brønd, Søren Brage, Peter Lund Kristensen, and Anders Grøntved. 2022. "Effects of Limiting Recreational Screen Media Use on Physical Activity and Sleep in Families with Children." *JAMA Pediatrics*, May. https://doi. org/10.1001/jamapediatrics.2022.1519.

14. Cleland, V, D Crawford, L A Baur, C Hume, A Timperio, and J Salmon. 2008. "A Prospective Examination of Children's Time Spent Outdoors, Objectively Measured Physical Activity and Overweight." /International Journal of Obesity/ 32 (11): 1685–93. https://doi.org/10.1038/ijo.2008.171; Kwon, Soyang, Pooja S. Tandon, Meghan E. O'Neill, and Adam B. Becker. 2022. "Cross-Sectional Association of Light Sensor-Measured Time Outdoors with Physical Activity and Gross Motor Competency among U.S. Preschool-Aged Children: The 2012 NHANES National Youth Fitness Survey." /BMC Public Health/ 22 (1). https://doi.org/10.1186/s12889-022-13239-0.

15. DeVos, Jody, 2022. "Why 'Opting Outside' Matters | Psychology Today." n.d. Www.psychologytoday.com. Accessed October 28, 2022. https://www.psychologytoday.com/us/blog/the-science-play/202210/why-opting-outside-matters.

16. Ellyn Satter Institute. "Your Child Will Naturally Be as Active as Is Right for Her." Accessed October 3, 2022. https://www.ellynsatterinstitute.org/how-to-feed/the-division-of-responsibility-in-activity/; © Copyright 2022 by Ellyn Satter published at EllynSatterInstitute.org.

17. Rennung, Miriam, and Anja S. Göritz. 2016. "Prosocial Consequences of Interpersonal Synchrony." *Zeitschrift Für Psychologie* 224 (3): 168–89. https://doi.org/10.1027/2151-2604/a000252; Mogan, Reneeta, Ronald Fischer, and Joseph A. Bulbulia. 2017. "To Be in Synchrony or Not? A Meta-Analysis of Synchrony's Effects on Behavior, Perception, Cognition and Affect." *Journal of Experimental Social Psychology* 72 (September): 13–20. https://doi.org/10.1016/j.jesp.2017.03.009;

18. Anderson, Elizabeth, and Geetha Shivakumar. "Effects of Exercise and Physical Activity on Anxiety." Frontiers in Psychiatry 4 (April 23, 2013): 27. https://doi.org/10.3389/fpsyt.2013.00027.

19. Christophe André. 2019. 'Proper Breathing Brings Better Health " Scientific American. January 15, 2019. https://www.scientificamerican.com/article/proper-breathing-brings-better-health/.

20. "Yoga and Body Image: How Do Young Adults Practicing Yoga Describe Its Impact on Their Body Image?" Body Image 27 (December 1, 2018): 156–68. https://doi.org/10.1016/j.bodyim.2018.09.001;

21. Eime, Rochelle M., Janet A. Young, Jack T. Harvey, Melanie J. Charity, and Warren R. Payne. "A Systematic Review of the Psychological and Social Benefits of Participation in Sport for Children and Adolescents: Informing Development of a Conceptual Model of Health through Sport."

International Journal of Behavioral Nutrition and Physical Activity 10, no. 1 (August 15, 2013): 98. https://doi.org/10.1186/1479-5868-10-98.

CHAPTER TEN: BODY

1. Piran, N. New possibilities in the prevention of eating disorders: The introduction of positive body image measures. Body Image (2015), http://dx.doi.org/10.1016/j.bodyim.2015.03.008

2. Tantleff-Dunn, et al., "It's Not Just a 'Woman Thing:' The Current State of Normative Discontent."

3. Lowes, Jacinta, and Marika Tiggemann. 2003. "Body Dissatisfaction, Dieting Awareness and the Impact of Parental Influence in Young Children." /British Journal of Health Psychology/ 8 (2): 135–47. https://doi.org/10.1348/135910703321649123; Jones, Chelsea C., and Stacy L. Young. 2021. "The Mother-Daughter Body Image Connection: The Perceived Role of Mothers' Thoughts, Words, and Actions." /Journal of Family Communication/, March, 1–9. https://doi.org/10.1080/15267431.2021.1908294; "Influence of Mothers on the Development of Body Dissatisfaction in Daughters in Daughters." n.d. Accessed December 17, 2020. https://scholarsarchive.byu.edu/cgi/viewcontent.cgi?article=1025&context=intuition.

4. Vuong, An T., Hannah K. Jarman, Jo R. Doley, and Siân A. McLean. 2021. "Social Media Use and Body Dissatisfaction in Adolescents: The Moderating Role of Thin- and Muscular-Ideal Internalisation." International Journal of Environmental Research and Public Health 18 (24): 13222. https://doi.org/10.3390/ijerph182413222; Jiotsa, Barbara, Benjamin Naccache, Mélanie Duval, Bruno Rocher, and Marie Grall-Bronnec. 2021. "Social Media Use and Body Image Disorders: Association between Frequency of Comparing One's Own Physical Appearance to that of People Being Followed on Social Media and Body Dissatisfaction and Drive for Thinness." International Journal of Environmental Research and Public Health 18 (6): 2880. https://doi.org/10.3390/ijerph18062880; Kelly, Yvonne, Afshin Zilanawala, Cara Booker, and Amanda Sacker. 2019. "Social Media Use and Adolescent Mental Health: Findings from the UK Millennium Cohort Study." EClinicalMedicine 6 (2589-5370): 59–68. https://doi.org/10.1016/j.eclinm.2018.12.005; Hunt, Melissa G., Rachel Marx, Courtney Lipson, and Jordyn Young. 2018. "No More FOMO: Limiting Social Media Decreases Loneliness and Depression." Journal of Social and Clinical Psychology 37 (10): 751–68. https://doi.org/10.1521/jscp.2018.37.10.751.

5. Snapp, Shannon, Laura Hensley-Choate, and Ehri Ryu. "A Body Image Resilience Model for First-Year College Women." Sex Roles 67, no. 3 (August 1, 2012): 211–21. https://doi.org/10.1007/s11199-012-0163-1.

ABOUT THE AUTHOR

Amelia Sherry, MPH, RD, CDN, CDCES, is a registered and certified dietitian nutritionist, a certified diabetes care and education specialist, and has been writing about women's health and nutrition since her first job at *American Health* magazine in 1999. She is also the founder of NourishHer, an online resource hub that offers women and girls alternative ways to think about nutrition so they can live happier, healthier lives. Through her private practice, teaching, speaking, and writing, she advocates for non-diet approaches to eating and wellness for people across the weight spectrum. To take part in a workshop and learn more about the positive food parenting strategies she teaches, visit NourishHer.com or follow her on Instagram @ ameliasherryRD.

Did you like this book? If so, please consider sharing it. Your recommendation is a vitally important kind of social currency that no amount of marketing or publicity I do can ever replace. You can write a review on Amazon.com, Barnesandnoble.com Bookshop.org., or Goodreads.com, sharing the book on social media, or simply mention it to another mother. You can also ask your local library to order *Diet-Proof Your Daughter* (and other non-diet titles you love!) for their collection, which can help spread these messages to other mothers in your community. Sending you a giant thank you for all you do (seen and unseen) to bring more good into the world for girls.

www.ingramcontent.com/pod-product-compliance
Lightning Source LLC
Chambersburg PA
CBHW030406130626
46549CB00004B/1658